Champneys

A-Z GUIDE TO
POSITIVE HEALTH

Editor CHRISTINE AZIZ

Published by Harmsworth Publications Ltd.,
for Associated Newspapers plc,
Carmelite House, London EC4Y 0JA.

ISBN 0 85144 513 6

Acknowledgments

Dianne Allwood CIDESCO FSBTh
Spa Manager

Paula Gilbert SRD
Dietician

Amanda Rashid RGN ONC
Senior Sister

Pam Wells SRN
Sister

Sue Sims RGN
Assistant Manager

Dr Colin Crosby BA MA MB BS LRCP MRCS
Medical Adviser

Ellen Pratley SRN ABEOA Reg ACUP
Osteopath

David Barton BSc (Physiotherapy)
Physiotherapist

John Lavan BA (Sports Studies)
Senior Exercise Instructor

Candace Johnston BA (Hons)
Lifestyle Consultant

Rosalie Pyatt
Senior Stylist

Dr Zena Maxwell MBChB
Champneys College Director

Anne Murray BABTAC
Champneys College Principal

Angela Brackley ITEC
Assistant Spa Manager

Typesetting by I. C. Dawkins
(Typesetters), London EC1.
Colour separation by Mullis
Morgan, London WC1.
Printed by William Clowes Ltd.,
Beccles, Suffolk.

Book designed by Ceri Weeks.

Cover picture by Clive Arrowsmith

CONTENTS

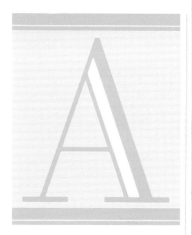

A

ABDOMEN

Some people call it the belly, others the stomach but it's really the abdomen. It lies below the chest and above the pelvis. Its roof is dome-shaped muscle called the diaphragm and it extends down into the pelvis, the floor of which consists of an overlapping muscular sheet. The upper part is enclosed by ribs and is protected behind the backbone by muscle on either side.

The abdominal wall is made up of thin sheets of muscle covered with fat and skin on its front and sides. It expands to accommodate breathing, pregnancy and eating. The kidneys, bladder, adrenal glands, liver, spleen and part of the digestive tract including the stomach, are all contained within the abdomen. It is lined with a slippery membrane called the peritoneum, which allows the organs to slide easily on one another and against the abdomen wall as they move during breathing and digestion.

A strong abdomen not only keeps the major organs in position, but also supports the back. (Slack abdominal muscles allow the pelvis to slip forward, creating strain on the back muscles and lower spine.) It can also be an indicator of how efficiently you are breathing; it's the abdomen, not your chest, that should expand as you breathe in. (See BREATHING, MEDITATION, RELAXATION.)

Exercises to strengthen stomach muscles are essential after pregnancy or sudden weight loss, when they have been under severe strain and are most in need of toning and strengthening.

Swimming, aerobics, belly dancing and fixed weight training are all good ways of firming up a neglected abdomen.

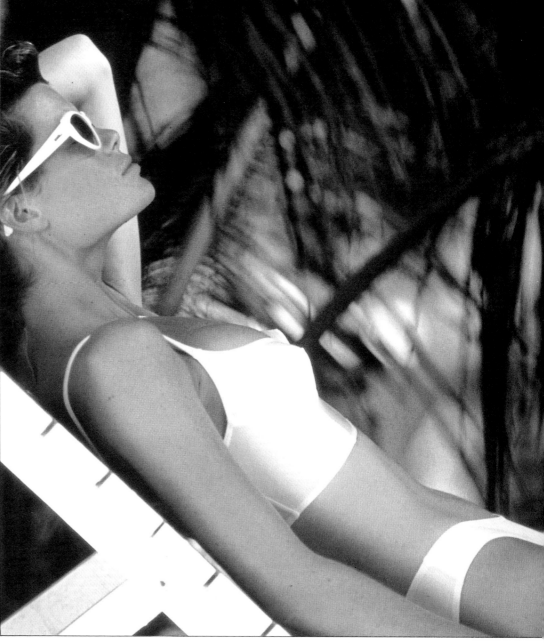

Why not try these two exercises at home each day? At the end of four weeks your muscles won't feel like sponge any more!
- Lie on your back
Bring knees up to chest
Cross your ankles and half-straighten legs
Curl head and shoulders up and draw pelvic bone towards you. Lift up tailbone slightly
Make sure your abdominal muscles are doing the work and not your neck
Check that your abdomen pulls in and down
Half-uncurl and repeat ten times.
- Sitting, rest back on elbows, with shoulders down
Pull abdominal muscles in so that your back presses down. Feel it touching the floor
Bend and straighten alternate legs
Repeat 20 to 30 times.

ACNE

Acne affects mainly teenagers but can affect adults too. The sebaceous glands produce an oil called sebum which lubricates skin and hair. During puberty these glands increase in size and produce extra sebum that can obstruct the pores, attracting bacteria and infecting the sebaceous glands. As a result blackheads, whiteheads, pimples and ugly red and purple lumps appear.

In adults acne is usually caused by an imbalance of the sex hormones testosterone and progesterone. Stress, early pregnancy, the contraceptive pill and onset of menstruation can all trigger acne. It can also be an allergic reaction.

It is important to treat acne in the early stages – as soon as the first blackheads and whiteheads are noticed. Serious advanced acne can cause emotional and psychological problems as well as scarring.

Overhaul your diet: avoid fatty meats, highly processed foods, nuts, fried foods, chocolate, cocoa, iodised salt and shellfish. Eat plenty of fresh fruit, raw vegetables, garlic and watercress and foods rich in vitamin A (fish, liver, eggs, fish roe) and zinc (meat, wholegrains). Switch from saturated fats (animal and coconut fats) to unsaturated (vegetable, corn and sunflower oils).
Treatments include…
- Extra vitamins: excess sebum is reduced by riboflavin (B2) and pyridoxine (B6). Infection may be prevented by vitamin C (between six to eight grams a·day). Prevent scarring with vitamin E taken in capsule form or as an oil rubbed over

● Antibiotic tablets: these can only be prescribed by your doctor. The antibiotics most often prescribed are tetracyclines, which can cause yeast type vaginal infections and shouldn't be taken during pregnancy.

Other suitable antibiotics include erythromycin, ampicillin and clindamycin.

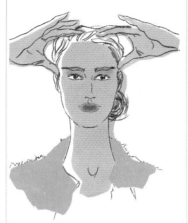

ACUPRESSURE

Points on the meridians (see ACUPUNCTURE) called tsubos are pressed by the fingertips only for a specific number of seconds to stimulate or sedate energy flows. The tsubos are acupuncture points and when gently pressed can quickly relieve headaches, stress and muscular pains. For example, light pressure on the temple with a gentle rotating movement can relieve headaches caused by facial tension. (See SHIATSU.)

ACUPUNCTURE

Acupuncture is a traditional Chinese medicine based on an invisible system of 14 energy channels known as meridians. An imbalance in these natural energies produces illness. To restore balance, needles are inserted into acupuncture points which tap into the meridians, reducing or increasing energy levels.

There are at least 2,000 acupuncture points, and the meridians flow through the organs, nerves, brain, skin and respiratory system. Apart from the central and governing meridians, all the channels are bilateral. Yin meridians run from the toes upwards and Yang meridians run from the head and fingertips. Each pair is governed by the five elements: fire, earth, metal, water and wood.

The interplay of these forces is believed to create the energy for life.

The World Health Organisation has compiled a list of medical conditions which respond well to acupuncture. They include: asthma; neurological and musculoskeletal disorders such as low back pain and headaches; digestive disorders such as gastritis and colitis; chronic menstrual problems; mental and emotional disturbances; addiction.

Acupuncture is also an effective anaesthetic, probably because the needles stimulate the release of endorphines – the brain's natural painkillers – or jam the central nervous system preventing pain signals reaching the brain.

The acupuncturist will try to locate the disharmony which underlies your problems by:
● Looking into your physical, emotional, spiritual and social life
● Examining your skin, the palms of your hands and tongue
● Feeling 12 meridian pulses – six in each wrist. Each relates to specific meridians and has a different quality such as slippery, rough, wiry
● Needles are then inserted into several acupuncture points considered most appropriate for treating your disharmony. The needles are made of steel, and are safe and painless. Occasionally there's a sensation like a mild electric shock. The needles are left in the skin for up to 20 minutes and can be stimulated by gentle agitation.

ADDITIVES

Food additives are chemical 'cocktails' used mainly to preserve, colour and flavour a wide range of goods. Most additives have no nutritional value and medical research has shown that additives are a common cause of allergies, hyperactivity and asthma in children. Many of these chemicals are not tested nor are they under the control of government departments. Only 60 per cent of the additives found in Britain's shops have been tested. Most pre-packed and convenience foods contain additives, although unpackaged fruit and vegetables may contain residues of artificial fertilisers and pesticides. Meat can contain hormones and antibiotics given to animals.

Food additives are known to affect health in three main ways:
● Carcinogenic – produce cancers
● Teratogenic – affect unborn children
● Mutagenic – stimulate changes in gene patterns, probably affecting future generations.

Public pressure has forced more retailers to offer a wider selection of foods free from artificial additives, preservatives and flavourings. Manufacturers are bound by law to list ingredients, and the safest bet is to read the contents label. But be warned, packaging can be misleading – that carton which says 'Free from artificial colours and flavouring' may include preservatives in the small print. Bread that boldly proclaims itself free from all artificial colours may still contain anti-oxidants.

The future use of additives is in the hands of the consumer. Manufacturers will only be forced to provide healthier alternatives if people refuse to buy goods containing food additives.
● Start by nagging local shopkeepers to carry a wider range of additive-free foods.
● Avoid highly processed packaged foods like instant trifles, whips and puddings. These are some of the worst offenders along with squash, fizzy drinks, brightly coloured sweets, lollipops, ice lollies. All of them are aimed at children.
● Become a label reader.

the area of infected skin.
● Skin hygiene: using clean hands, wash affected areas at least three times a day with mild soaps and warm water. After rinsing, splash with cold water to close pores.
● Skin lotions, gels and creams: the most effective treatments contain benzoyl peroxide and are available from the chemist under many brand names.
● Vitamin A lotions and gels contain retinoids, compounds of the vitamin, and help to loosen blackheads. Retinoic acid is a synthetic cousin of vitamin A and available only through dermatologists. It dramatically reduces sebum production and suppresses inflammation. If skin is severely infected, Resorcinol – a strong crystalline antiseptic soluble in water, alcohol and oils – may also be prescribed.

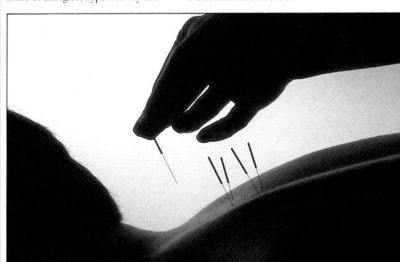

IAN BRADSHAW, TRANSWORLD, JACQUELINE BISSETT

AEROBICS

Aerobic exercise involves rhythmic movements of arms and legs and a contracting and stretching of large muscle groups. Regular aerobic exercise should put the body under measured steady stress to build stamina, strength, suppleness and endurance.

The aim of aerobics is to increase the amount of oxygen the body can process in a given time, ie the body's aerobic capacity; any EXERCISE that increases the heart rate and so pumps more blood around the body can be aerobic. Skipping, running, jogging, dance, swimming, cycling, walking and rowing are all aerobic exercises and fun to do.

Swimming is considered the most effective form of aerobic activity. It uses every major muscle group, has a low injury risk and – because water is weight bearing – is ideal for pregnant women and overweight people. For full benefit any aerobic activity must be sustained for a period of not less than 20 minutes – the recommendation is a minimum of three half-hour workouts per week.

The benefits are enormous…
- Energy and stamina increase
- Better sleeping habits – a deeper sleep
- Improved emotional state
- Improved circulation
- Relieves depression
- Can increase natural resistance to infection
- Provides protection against post-menopausal OSTEOPOROSIS.

If you have a history of back problems, high blood pressure, respiratory problems, chest pain, oedema (water retention), dizzy spells, or if you are recuperating from an illness, it is wise to consult your doctor before starting a new exercise programme.

Start exercising gently, and stop if you feel any pain or dizziness. You may like to take your PULSE once or twice while exercising to monitor your progress. After exercise the speed at which your pulse rate returns to normal is an indicator of your fitness level.

A rough guide to your maximum heartrate is arrived at by deducting your age from 220. Reduce this number by one quarter to work out your safe limit for your age during aerobic exercise – if you are 30, for example, a pulse rate of 145 is high enough.

Try to work up from 60 to 80 per cent of maximum heart rate as you become fitter and can tolerate more vigorous exercise.

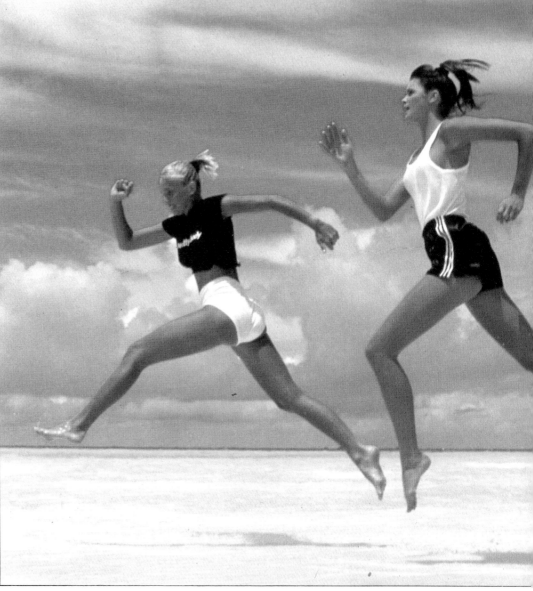

AGEING

Wisdom, peace and fulfilment are all part of the ageing process. The passage of time does not mean the inevitable loss of mental power, sexual potency, physical attractiveness and energy. How badly and quickly you age depends on your genetic inheritance, diet, stress, lifestyle, pollution and *you* – your own mental attitude.

The Hunzas in a remote area of Kashmir, the Vilcabamba Indians in the Andes and the Abkhazians in Soviet Georgia all live to a grand old age – some well into their hundreds. All three cultures have several things in common…
- They lead extremely active lives, regardless of age, and engage in physical labour every day.
- They are sexually active well into their 80s and 90s.
- They eat a low calorie diet – averaging 1,700 calories a day, compared to the daily British average of 3,000.
- Their diet is high in fresh foods, many eaten raw, and low in fats.
- They never eat sugar.
- The elderly are respected and valued within their communities.

It is possible to incorporate some of these factors into our lives…
- Cut down on calories and stick to a DIET that's rich in vitamins and minerals with plenty of fresh fruit and vegetables. Avoid alcohol and cigarettes. Cut down on coffee and tea. Restrict sugar to one ounce a day.
- We may not be able to work in the fields like the Hunzas, but we can halt the ageing effects of a sedentary lifestyle by taking up exercise. Regular AEROBIC activity can slow the ageing process by increasing heart output, lung capacity and blood volume. Oxygen nourishes our cells, but maximal oxygen volume decreases by one per cent per year. Moderate exercise in an older person can achieve the oxygen uptake of a

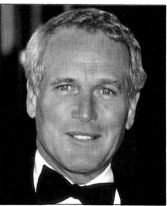

person 15 years younger. A very active person can achieve the uptake of a person 40 years younger. Ease into exercising gently, and consult a doctor if you need to before you start.
- It is said that lovemaking is like wine – it gets better as you get older. Experience and a shift of emphasis to friendship and companionship in relationships can enhance sex in later years. Growing together in a

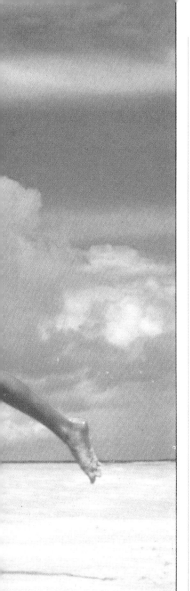

relationship gives a fuller, deeper sense of love. Making love not only relieves physical tension, but is also a means of emotional, physical and spiritual expression and should continue long after the first bloom of youth has faded. (See SEX.)
● Change attitudes! Psychologists have found that the changes in our bodies and minds associated with ageing can be determined by our 'programmed expectations'; if it is assumed that middle-age spread is inevitable at 40, it is likely to happen. A positive attitude to life and age is a key factor in staying youthful. This is best reflected in LAUGHTER. Research has shown that the more we laugh, the longer we live.

Look for positive role models, men and women who take obvious delight in their maturity – for example, Paul Newman (left), Audrey Hepburn, Rudolph Nureyev and Margaret Thatcher all prove that life really does begin after 40. (See POSITIVE THINKING.)

AIDS

Aids (Acquired Immune Deficiency Syndrome) is caused by a virus called Human Immunodeficiency Virus, or HIV. It attacks cells that normally defend the body from infection, until eventually the body can be taken over by a variety of fatal illnesses, known collectively as Aids. These include pneumonia, hepatitis, tuberculosis and rare cancers. There is no single definitive test for Aids. Instead blood is tested for HIV antibodies.

Aids is not highly contagious like colds or measles. HIV is transmitted in blood and sexual fluids – semen or vaginal – mainly through all forms of unprotected sexual intercourse (anal and vaginal), contact with infected blood, and by infected body fluids entering wounds. Or, during pregnancy, from mother to child.
PREVENTION
● Avoid penetrative sex and activities in which bodily fluids are exchanged.
● If you have penetrative sex always use a condom, preferably with spermicide containing nonoxynol – 9. Check that condoms meet the British Standard, BS 3704.
● Don't share needles and syringes.
● Worried? If you think you or your partner(s) have been exposed to the virus, contact your local Aidsline or the National Aids Helpline (see address list).
● You do need sympathetic support to consider how you wish to respond before you take any action. It is best to be careful about who you choose to discuss your anxieties with because of the high level of prejudice against anyone associated with HIV or Aids.

Many insurance companies are now asking whether or not applicants have ever sought treatment for a sexually transmitted disease. (See HIV, SAFE SEX.)

ALCOHOL

Alcohol is a depressant, dulling the brain and nervous system. In moderation alcohol can be beneficial – studies show that a very small amount can provide protection against heart disease. In large regular doses it can affect the co-ordination of muscles and nerves, impair vision, judgment and memory, weaken the body's immune system, cause sexual impotence by reducing quantities of the male sex hormone testosterone in the liver. It can also deplete vitamins,

especially thiamin (vitamin B_1).

Excessive consumption of alcohol can also kill – an increasing number of people are dying from cirrhosis of the liver and in road accidents caused by drunk drivers.

But how much alcohol can be consumed without risk to health and life? The medical profession recommends that men should drink no more than 21 units a week (a unit is equivalent to a glass of wine or half a pint of beer/lager or a single tot of spirits), and women 14 units.

These amounts should not be in binges, but spread over the whole week. Aim to have two or three alcohol-free days per week.

It is very easy to exceed these recommended limits if drinking is tied up with work and socialising: increasingly men and women are slipping into the regular habit of drinking at a working lunch, then drinking again in the evening to relax. (See RELAXATION.)

The liver can process a maximum of 80g of alcohol for a man (four pints of beer or a bottle of wine) and 40g for a woman within 24 hours, but will take 72 hours to return to normal. Taken regularly in these quantities alcohol can do irreparable liver damage.

To reduce your alcohol intake, try ordering a bottle of mineral water instead of a bottle of wine to accompany that working lunch. And always have a glass of mineral water alongside your alcoholic drink, or turn that glass of wine into a spritzer by adding mineral water.

The most effective way to beat a hangover is to drink lots of water before you go to bed. If you drink alcohol regularly you may need to supplement your diet with vitamins B and C. If alcohol is adversely affecting the quality of your life and loved ones, you may be dependent on it, and should seek professional help.

ALEXANDER TECHNIQUE

The failing voice of an Australian actor in the early 1900s led to the development of the Alexander Technique.

Frederick Matthias Alexander embarked on a long period of self-observation in order to discover the reason for his sudden hoarseness. But what at first seemed a problem with his voice apparently involved the muscular patterns of excessive tension throughout his whole body.

He developed a form of gentle guidance with his hands to reorganise muscle patterns in his friends. After

several visits to Alexander they found their health improved, as well as voice and breathing. Depression and anxieties lifted.

The Alexander Technique is a process of physical re-education, changing the way the body is used. Its aim is to improve 'the use of the self' by consciously avoiding harmful tensions, and encouraging more

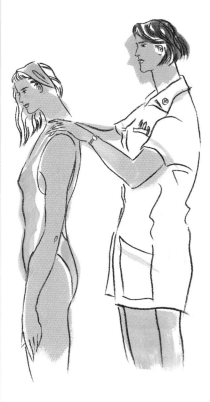

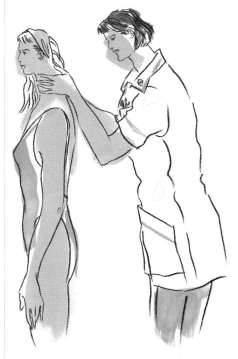

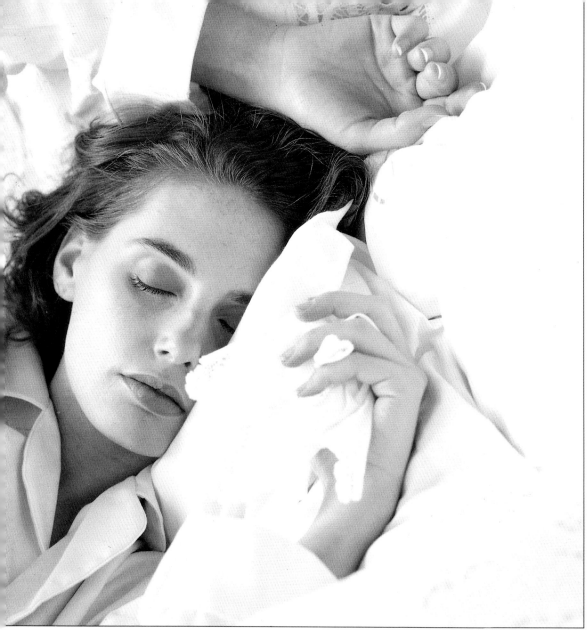

St Thomas's Hospital in London indicate that the most common allergens are cows' milk, eggs, wheat, artificial colourings, cheese, yeast and fish. Other common allergens include the contraceptive pill, gases, sprays, antibiotics and synthetic hormone residues in meat.

Some allergies can be easy to diagnose. For instance, if you only feel ill when you are at work, you may be suffering from Office Building Syndrome caused mainly by air conditioning. If you wake up every morning with the snuffles, it could be a pillow allergy.

Less obvious food allergies or intolerances can be diagnosed by rigidly following an exclusion diet for a set period under the supervision of a competent dietician or NATUROPATH. Bear these points in mind and take expert medical advice. . .

● Choose a time when commitments are minimal.

● The Food and Chemical Allergy Association recommends an elimination diet containing only the following: fresh lamb, fresh plaice, fresh pears, fresh cabbage, bottled mineral water (for drinking and cooking), sea salt.

● At the end of two weeks you will probably be advised to reintroduce foods daily. Note any obvious reactions.

● Start by introducing tap water and foods that are least likely to cause problems such as fruit, vegetables (except potatoes, peas and beans) and meat (except pork).

● Eat only small quantities and take only one in each 24-hour period as reaction may be delayed.

natural posture and movement patterns.

The teacher works on a one to one basis and gently detects hidden tensions and distorted muscles. Simple everyday movements are used to illustrate how to move with minimal tension. Each lesson lasts 30 to 40 minutes and an average of 25 lessons are needed for full benefit.

The teacher will begin with the neck and head. According to Alexander, neck movement in most people is inhibited by wrongly distributed muscle tension. As a result blood flow to the brain and breathing can be restricted.

The technique is unique in that it teaches you to stop making unnecessary effort in all kinds of different situations and you become more aware of balance, posture and movement in your daily activities.

The effects of Alexander's teaching have proved to be far reaching – although it is not yet known why. Improvements have been reported in various physical ailments including eczema, rheumatoid arthritis, headaches and spastic colon following a course in AT. Alexander students also report much greater mental and emotional well-being.

ALLERGIES

The word allergy is derived from Greek meaning 'altered reaction – this is exactly what an allergy is. Exposure to certain substances either in food or in the environment can provoke mental and physical symptoms in some individuals and may even cause or aggravate conditions such as eczema, catarrh, sinusitis, arthritis and hay fever. Fifty years ago a relatively small number of people were allergic, mainly to pollens, house dust mites and moulds. But the increase in the number of man-made chemical substances encountered in our daily lives – including pesticides, herbicides and artificial colourings – has led to an increase in sufferers. Eighty per cent of the UK population is now believed to be allergic to something.

Symptoms of allergy vary and can include visual disturbances, itching eyes, runny nose, sneezing, catarrh, ringing ears, cramps, abnormal heartbeat, lethargy, extremes of temperature, shaking, vaginal discharge, clumsiness, migraine, epilepsy, forgetfulness, depression, aggressiveness, arthritic joints.

Anyone can be allergic to anything, but there are certain foods and drinks which have higher allergenic properties than others. Studies at

ALTERNATIVE THERAPIES

Alternative therapies, or complementary medicine, can be divided into two main categories:

● Medicinal therapies – something taken by mouth as in HOMOEOPATHY, or applied to the skin as in AROMATHERAPY

● Body-mind therapies – these use the power of the mind to sustain good health and heal, as in MEDITATION and AUTOGENICS training. They also include physical treatment methods such as OSTEOPATHY and ROLFING.

Some therapies are complete health systems in their own right, such as NATUROPATHY, while others, such as HERBALISM, can be used in conjunction with other treatments.

Complementary practitioners consider health as a vibrant, positive state of wholeness, harmony and

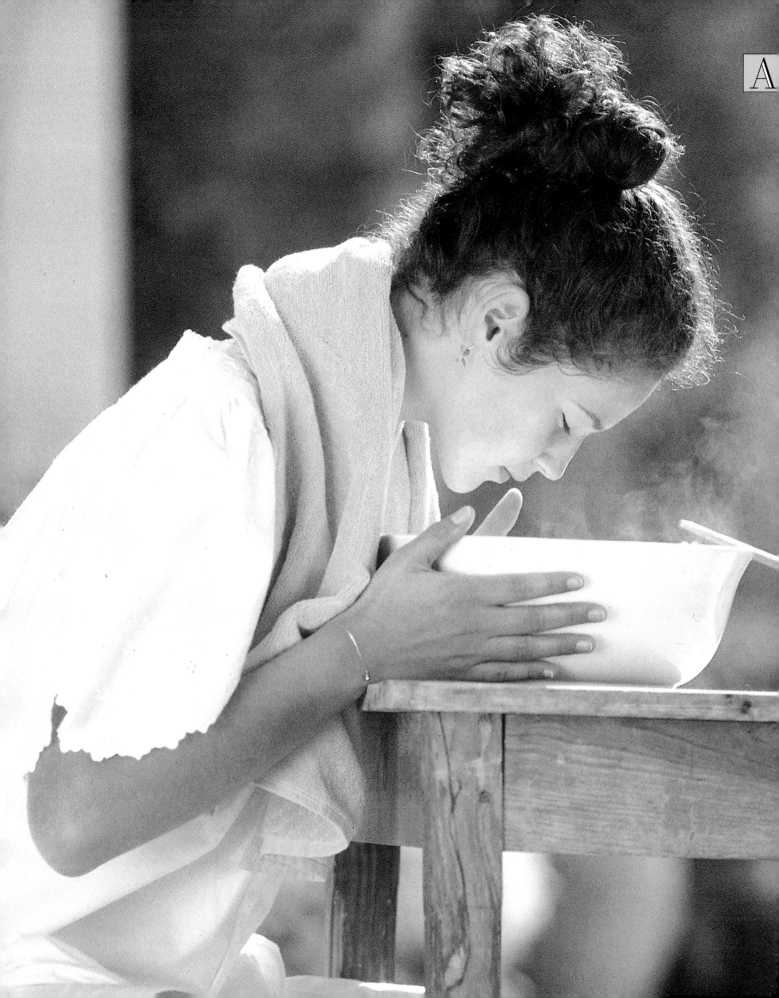

balance. Excessive stress or toxins in the body are believed to underlie all sickness, throwing the body out of balance. Symptoms of disease, such as nausea, sore throats, fever, are seen as the body's attempts to deal with imbalance and are a useful guideline to the nature of that imbalance. Most complementary medicines aim to treat the patient by…
● Strengthening the body's defences
● Unblocking energy flows
● Eliminating toxins
● Facilitating self-healing
● Treating the whole person.

In the last 20 years complementary medicine has become more popular in Britain, thanks largely to the Royal Family who often consult a homoeopath when ill.

A survey of 28,000 people by the Consumers Association revealed that one in seven respondents had consulted a complementary practitioner. The most widely used was osteopathy followed by homoeopathy. Many of the therapies have been in use for thousands of years – acupuncture, for instance, has been practised by the Chinese for 6,000 years. Others are more recent: the ALEXANDER TECHNIQUE and Autogenics were both developed early this century.

There is very little scientific evidence to prove one way or another the effectiveness of alternative therapies. Their effectiveness can only be measured by consumer satisfaction; out of every ten people who have used homoeopathy, seven said they would do so again.

Before consulting a complementary practitioner, check that he or she holds a qualification recognised by the therapy's professional body and is registered with that organisation.

AMINO ACIDS

Amino acids are chemical building blocks that make up protein – the main ingredient of our body cells. There are are 22 amino acids, but eight of these are called essential amino acids because we must get them from our diet, unlike the remaining amino acids which are produced by the body. The essential amino acids are isoleucine, leucine, lysine, methionine, phenylalanine, threonine, tryptophan and valine.

Most of the amino acids have specific functions, ranging from pain killing to sperm mobility and sleep enhancement.

Beans, meat, fish, eggs, dairy products and poultry all contain significant quantities of amino acids. But amino acids are often destroyed during cooking, although substances that inhibit digestion of amino acids remain in beans, including soya, if they are not thoroughly cooked.

The World Health Organisation recommends a protein intake of up to 37g per day during pregnancy. This should be enough to ensure a healthy intake of amino acids. However, in certain diseases and at certain times of life the demand for amino acids can increase. Amino acid supplements are increasingly being used to treat certain conditions – for example, lysine is used for recurrent cold sores and herpes infections; tryptophan has been used for the treatment of depression, particularly when insomnia is a symptom; isoleucine, leucine and valine are used to treat some liver complaints.

ANAEROBIC EXERCISE

Anaerobic exercise involves a high level of effort sustained over a short period of time. The aim is to use up more oxygen than the body takes in. Anaerobic activity, such as short sprints or gymnastics, develops muscle tone and power and enables the body to eventually produce bursts of strength and energy, but does not on its own produce overall fitness. (See EXERCISE, AEROBICS, FITNESS.)

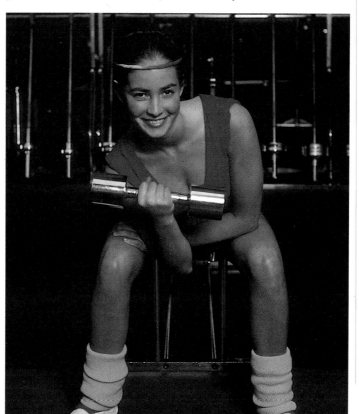

ANOREXIA NERVOSA

Anorexics suffer extreme weight loss by starving themselves. It is a condition that mainly affects women.

Distorted perceptions and low self-esteem lie at the heart of the anorexic's problem. Even when the sufferer looks emaciated they will see themselves as fat and overweight.

Psychologists believe anorexia nervosa is rooted in…
● A need to feel in control within the family unit, particularly with the mother. Sufferers are usually high achievers with high expectations
● Media promotion of 'thin is beautiful' image
● Constant thoughtless remarks that can plummet a teenager into a downward spiral of inadequacy.

It is possible to spot the symptoms fairly early on. Aside from drastic weight loss, look for…
● Swelling of the stomach, face and ankles
● Severe constipation
● Low blood pressure, resulting in extreme sensitivity to the cold
● An obsession with keeping fit
● Poor circulation – skin has a rough, discoloured appearance
● Impaired co-ordination
● Loss of hair.

Hospital treatment often involves two or three months on anti-depressants, under close supervision.

Force feeding is being replaced with an emphasis on nutritional

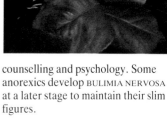

counselling and psychology. Some anorexics develop BULIMIA NERVOSA at a later stage to maintain their slim figures.

APHRODISIACS

For centuries men and women have been concocting potions that they hope will enhance and prolong sexual activity.

Nostradamus, the 16th-century astrologer, recommended a recipe that included mandrake root, the blood of male sparrows, tentacles of squid, musk, cloves, honey and Cretan wine. Good if you can get it!

Shellfish is said to promote virility because of the resemblance of the

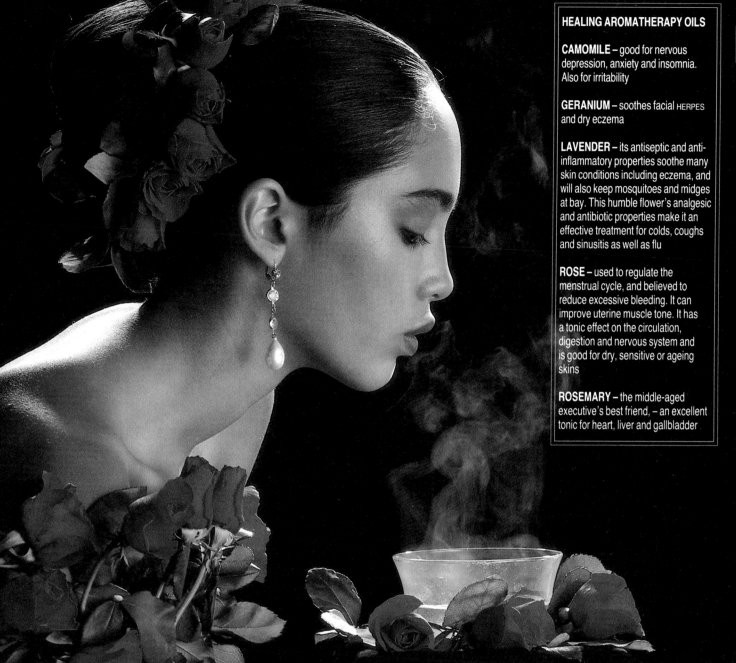

HEALING AROMATHERAPY OILS

CAMOMILE – good for nervous depression, anxiety and insomnia. Also for irritability

GERANIUM – soothes facial HERPES and dry eczema

LAVENDER – its antiseptic and anti-inflammatory properties soothe many skin conditions including eczema, and will also keep mosquitoes and midges at bay. This humble flower's analgesic and antibiotic properties make it an effective treatment for colds, coughs and sinusitis as well as flu

ROSE – used to regulate the menstrual cycle, and believed to reduce excessive bleeding. It can improve uterine muscle tone. It has a tonic effect on the circulation, digestion and nervous system and is good for dry, sensitive or ageing skins

ROSEMARY – the middle-aged executive's best friend, – an excellent tonic for heart, liver and gallbladder.

mollusc to female genitals. Celery is reputed to be the main ingredient of the love potion drunk by Tristan and Isolde. Mint is a popular aphrodisiac in the Middle East and the vibrant nasturtium is sometimes called the 'love flower' because of its reputation for arousing remarkable passion. Certain ESSENTIAL OILS are also believed to be aphrodisiacs.

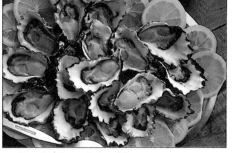

An aphrodisiac alone will not revive an ailing love life, but you may enjoy the fun of trying one.

A loss of libido can be caused by ill health, stress, overwork, a poor diet or a lack of love and communication in a relationship.

Lack of sexual enjoyment and appetite can also indicate low self-esteem or fear of pregnancy or intimacy itself.

If there are problems ignoring them will make things worse, so consult a doctor, complementary practitioner and/or a sex therapist.

AROMATHERAPY

The ancient healing art of aromatherapy uses oils extracted from plants, leaves, bark, roots, seeds and resins to treat a wide range of ailments, stress and emotional upset. For greatest therapeutic effect ESSENTIAL OILS are diluted in a carrier oil such as olive, almond or wheatgerm, and massaged into the skin. They can also be inhaled (see STEAM) and used in the bath. They are never taken internally and should only be applied undiluted to the skin by, or in consultation with, a qualified aromatherapist.

Research at the Instituto Derivato Vegetali in Milan shows that certain essential oils including jasmine and basil can dispel general depression. It is still not known how the essential oils work, but it is known that the thousands of tiny nerve cells in the nose contain odour molecules. The nerves themselves are connected to the part of the brain concerned with emotional drives, creativity and sexual behaviour. This could explain why some perfumes make us happy, why some, like rose, work as an aphrodisiac and why unpleasant smells like petrol can trigger depression. The oils also affect the body's hormone-producing glands and are known to remain longer in an ailing organ than a healthy one.

Store the oils in a cool place, but not in the fridge – low temperatures destroy the odoriferous molecules. For massage, use a three per cent concentration of essential oil to carrier oil.

concentration of essential oil to carrier oil.

Essential oils should not be used without first consulting a well trained aromatherapist. Certain essential oils have harmful side effects: basil, hyssop and myrrh should not be used in pregnancy; sage and thyme should be avoided by anyone suffering from high blood pressure. Sage and aniseed are the most toxic of all and can damage the nervous system. Epileptics should never use sage, fennel, hyssop or wormwood.

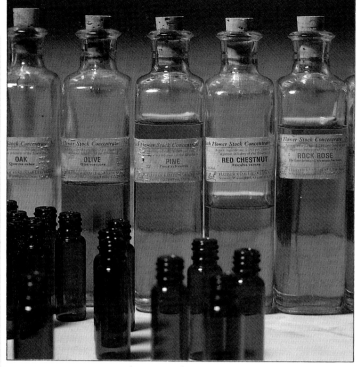

AUTOGENICS

The literal meaning of autogenics is 'generated from within'. A series of simple mental exercises combining autosuggestion with meditation techniques, autogenics is believed to combat stress and promote self-healing by inducing deep relaxation. The mental exercises were developed in the 1930s by German psychiatrist Johannes H Schultz.

Autogenics requires expert tuition and can be taught in groups or individually. The method concentrates on acquiring the skill to focus inwardly and encourage deep psycho-physical relaxation; the exercises are aimed to produce sensations of heaviness and warmth in the legs, regulate the heartbeat and breathing, induce abdominal warmth and cool the forehead. Unlike Eastern meditation techniques, autogenics can be learned quickly, and the benefits are similar.

The basic exercises are very simple but need to be practised daily. In a quiet room, wearing loose, comfortable clothes, either lie on your back with arms to the side or sit slumped on a stool, or lounge in an armchair. Close your eyes and focus on your arms. Repeat 'My arms are heavy' several times, and move on to your legs and the heart, 'My heart-beat is regular and calm'. Work through the body until you feel profoundly relaxed. Cancel the training session by clenching your hands and bringing them sharply up with a deep breath. Stretch.

Used by many professional athletes to reduce anxiety in competition, autogenics shares the health benefits of regular exercise such as lowered resting-heart beat and reduced high blood pressure, as well as providing a greater improvement in mental well-being. Advanced techniques can be used to help deep-rooted anxieties and disorders.

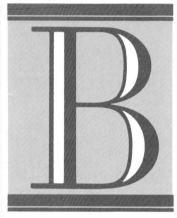

BACH FLOWER REMEDIES

Bach flower remedies do not deal with physical disorders, but their devotees believe they treat emotional disorders that underlie so many physical ailments.

In the 1920s a London doctor, Edward Bach, classified people into personality archetypes, each with a habitual negative emotional state such as indecision or fear. He selected plants, known as the Twelve Healers, which he believed would transform these emotions into positive ones, and went on to discover 26 other plant remedies known as The Helpers.

The Bach remedies can be bought in health food stores or homoeopathic pharmacies. It is not known how the remedies work, but Dr Bach's disciples suggest that particular plants of particular colours have patterns of vibration that can be transmitted to sunlit and heated water.

Dosage: take four drops of a chosen remedy in a little spring water four times a day for a month, on an empty stomach. The Bach Rescue Remedy, also available over the counter, is a treatment for shock. It contains star of Bethlehem, cherry plum, rock roses and clematis and may be taken as often as required.

The treatments are cheap to buy and finely balanced, but if you want to tune into flowers at home you can.
1 Take a ½ pt thin glass bowl.
2 Fill with pure water – not distilled. Mineral or spring water will do.
3 Pick the blossoms from the plant and float immediately on the water.
4 Cover the bowl and place in the sunshine, or heat gently.
5 Using a twig of the plant, lift blooms from the water.
6 Pour essence into clean bottles, adding an equal measure of brandy as preservative.
Store in a cool, dark place.

THE TWELVE HEALERS

MIMULUS – fear
CERATO – self distrust
ROCK ROSE – terror
SCLERANTHUS – indecision
GENTIAN – despondency
CLEMATIS – dreaminess
WATER VIOLET – excessive self-sufficiency
AGRIMONY – concealed worries
CENTAURY – the inability to say no, lack of assertiveness
CHICORY – tendency to take over
IMPATIENS – impatience
VERVAIN – over-enthusiasm

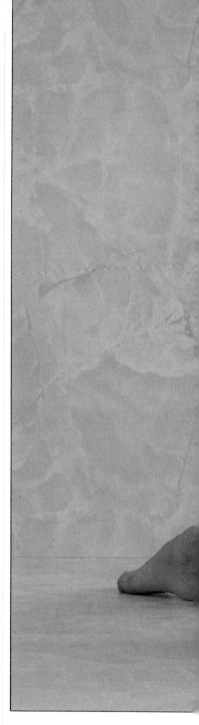

BACK

The back is a wonderful example of nature's engineering skills. The spine is the axis, anchor and load bearer. Muscles, joints, ligaments, cartilages and tendons work together as a harmonious whole, co-ordinating the mechanics of movement and weight bearing. Limbs, ribs and skull also play a part in the smooth functioning of our backs; their muscles and ligaments interweave with their counterparts along the spine to maintain balance and continuity of

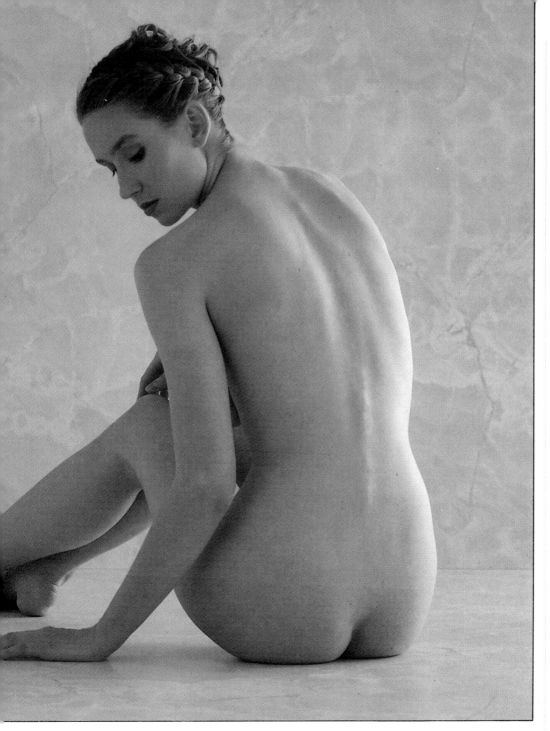

pelvis should tilt upwards and slightly forward, pushing the hollow of your back flat against the wall. With enough practice you will assume the posture naturally and your habitual posture will improve.

● *Are you sitting comfortably?*
Pressure on the spine is greatest when seated. Use straight-backed firm chairs with support just above the buttocks (the lumbar region). There should be suitable height adjustment. Sit with legs forward to minimise pressure behind the knee.
Don't slump or slouch forward. Knees should be level with or lower than hips.

● *Loosen up*
Clothes which restrict mobility of the hip and knees, such as tight jeans, can cause back pain. Also, avoid wearing high heels for long periods.

● *Bedtime*
Check the suitability of your bed by lying down and inserting hand between the bed and the small of your back. Your hand should be a snug fit. The bed is too soft if you can't do this easily. If your hand finds plenty of space, the bed is too hard.
When getting into bed lower body on to elbow and shoulder, draw up knees until feet are on the mattress then roll body over to face ceiling. Reverse these movements when getting out – bend both knees and don't leap up!

● *Lifting and carrying*
Carry objects as close to the body as possible. Use two lighter bags when shopping rather than one heavy bag. When lifting, stand close to the load, feet either side of the weight.
Keep back straight at all times.
Get down to the level of the load by bending hips and knees. With elbows close to the thighs grip the load, preferably with one hand below and to one side, the other above on the other side. With one smooth co-ordinated movement straighten the hips and knees, lifting the object close to the body. Reverse lifting action when lowering.

● *Drive in comfort*
Car seats generally have no support in the lumbar region, so fit a cushion or one of the many manufactured supports available. Adjust seat for maximum comfort so hips and knees are well flexed, with arms relaxed and bent to the driving wheel. On long journeys make regular stops and walk around. Try a few stretching exercises if possible. (See STRETCHING.)

● *Exercise*
Take up a safe non-weight-bearing exercise – swimming is ideal. YOGA and DANCE strengthen back and develop gracefulness.

movement. Four out of five people experience back pain at some time during their lives for a variety of reasons:
● A damaged or worn disc bulging under pressure presses against the ligaments of the spine which are very sensitive to pain.
● Nerve root pressure which can be caused by a ruptured disc pressing on the spinal nerves.
● Inflammation of the joints either through injury or an inflammatory condition such as some arthritis.
● Painful muscle spasm triggered by a number of stresses: poor posture, occupational hazards, bad seating,

unsuitable beds, injury or strain.
Speedy diagnosis and treatment are essential, so seek help rather than just waiting for back pain to ease. Back pain can be the symptom of a number of diseases affecting the gall stones, the kidneys, female reproductive organs and can indicate some types of cancer. These need to be ruled out before you decide which one of the many BACK-TREATMENTS you prefer, eg chartered physiotherapist, OSTEOPATHY, ACUPUNCTURE, CHIROPRACTIC, ALEXANDER TECHNIQUE, ROLFING.
Here are several preventative measures – all quite simple, but

particularly useful for keeping back pain at bay…

● Check posture
Poor posture puts stress on major weight-bearing joints such as ankles, pelvis and knees. Rounded shoulders or a hollow back increase stress on particular vertebrae. Improve posture by practising this exercise every day.
Stand tall against a wall and imagine you are being suspended from the top of your head by a piece of string. Keep head, shoulders, buttocks and heels in contact with the wall and tighten abdominal and buttock muscles. The front of your

BACK CARE EXERCISES

The following exercises give a general guide to mobilising and strengthening the spine. They will aid the prevention of back and neck pain. They may also be beneficial in long-standing or recurrent problems.

■ Safety
Certain precautions should be observed at all times while exercising to avoid causing strain or aggravating any problems. If you are experiencing either severe back pain, associated leg pain or your first bout of pain, it is important that you consult your doctor before undertaking back exercises.

Do not attempt to move 'through pain'. A slight pulling or stiffness is acceptable but anything more can be harmful.

If an exercise is making your pain worse stop that particular exercise.

If exercise in general is aggravating the pain cease performing all exercise and consult your practitioner.

■ Quality of Movement
Loose clothing should be worn so as not to restrict movements.

Allow a few minutes to relax fully, while lying down, before you begin. Deep breathing exercises are useful.

All exercises for the spine should be done slowly and in a controlled manner. Develop a clear sense of the feeling of each movement.

Be sure to continue breathing normally while performing any exercises. You may need to overcome a common tendency to hold your breath while concentrating on a particular movement. Abdominal and all other strengthening exercises should be performed co-ordinating the exhalation with the phase of exertion.

BACK FACTS
Back pain costs British industry £1,000 million in lost productivity each year

There's a one in two chance of back pain recurring

Each year 35 million working days are lost to backache

MOBILISING EXERCISES

▢ Stretch
Lying flat, take the left arm up above the head and stretch up and away with the left arm and down and away with the left hip and leg. Feel the stretch down the left side of the body, gently extending it as you exhale.
   Repeat slowly three times. Then repeat the exercise with the right arm and right leg.

▢ Pelvic tilt
Lying flat with the knees bent, keeping the feet on the floor – push the hollow of the back down on to the floor, then relax.
   Repeat six times.

▢ Unilateral hip flexion
Lying flat, bend up right knee and clasp hands around it. Squeeze gently towards the chest and relax.
   Repeat six times, then change to the left knee.

▢ Hump and hollow
Kneel on all fours. Firstly, arch the spine up towards the ceiling by tucking the head and bottom in and tightening the tummy muscles, then hollow the spine by looking up, pushing the bottom out and allowing the small of the back to sag downwards.
   Repeat slowly six times.

▢ Bilateral hip flexion
Lying flat, bend up both knees and clasp one hand around the front of each knee.
   Squeeze gently towards the chest and relax, allowing the knees to be held at arms' length.
   Keep the head on the floor during this exercise and repeat six times.

▢ Rotation
Lying flat, knees bent, feet on the floor, arms at right angles to the body, allow the knees to roll gently from side to side.
   Repeat six times to each side.

LOWER BACK

These exercises should be done in a standing position. They are designed to prevent and also relieve pain resulting from slouched sitting and bending or prolonged standing.

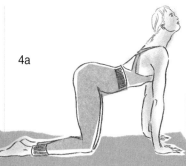

4a

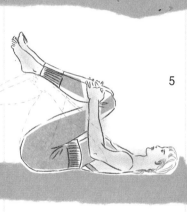

4b

5

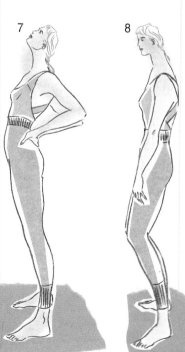

7   8

▢ Back arching
Place the hands in small of back and arch the upper part of the spine backwards. Relax back to the upright position.
   This is an invaluable exercise to interrupt or follow any forward bending movements or slouched sitting, as it reverts the strain occurring at the disc.
   Repeat four times.

▢ Pelvic tilt
Feet apart, bend knees slightly. Bring the front of the pelvis forward and upward by tightening the abdominal muscles at the front and tucking in the backside. The natural curve in the lower back will flatten as you do so. This reduces the compression at the back of the vertebrae and is therefore valuable in reducing the discomfort often associated with being in a static upright position for a prolonged period. Hold the position for three to four seconds.
   Repeat approximately four times every 15 minutes when having to stand for a long time.

ABDOMINAL EXERCISES

▢ Pelvic tilt
   As in exercise Number 2, but hold for three seconds.

▢ Head and shoulders lift
Lying flat, keeping the knees bent and feet on the floor, tilt the pelvis and tuck the chin on to the chest. Then lift the head and shoulders and run the fingers up to the knees. Hold for five seconds, then lower down and relax. Repeat six times. Feel the gentle curling movement of the spine.

▢ Isometric oblique
Lying flat, lift the right knee so that the thigh is vertical and place the left hand against the top of the knee – keep the knee still, but try to push it down towards the floor with the left hand. Repeat six times, then change to the left knee and right hand.

▢ Knee roll
Lie flat, then come up on to the elbows and bend the knees, keeping the feet on the floor. Tilt the pelvis and lift the knees up to the chest; gradually lower the legs until the feet

10

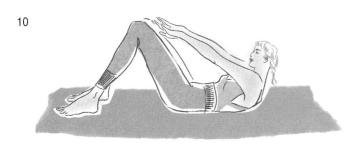

11

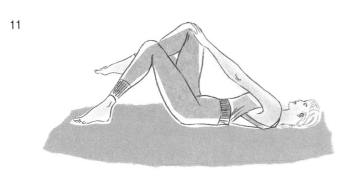

are *almost* touching the floor. Hold for five seconds and then bend up again. Be sure to keep the pelvis tilted and knees bent at all times.

NECK AND SHOULDERS

All these exercises are done in the sitting position.

13 Neck retraction
Allow the chin to jut forwards, then tuck the chin into the chest and stretch upwards with the crown of the head, attempting to lengthen the spine. Hold for two seconds, then relax.
Repeat four times.

14 Side flexion
Place the right hand on the left shoulder, then gently tilt the head sideways towards the right shoulder. Apply gentle pressure to the left shoulder with the hand and

feel a gradual stretch to the left side of the neck.
Repeat three times then change to the other side.

15 Rotation
Slowly turn the head to look over one shoulder, then slowly back to look over the other, keeping eyes straight ahead.
Repeat three times to each side.

16 Shoulder blade rotation
Place the hands on the shoulders, bring the elbows forwards, up, back and down in a circling movement. Co-ordinate the breathing during this exercise to breathe in as you are making the forwards and upwards movements and to breathe out during the backwards and downwards movements. Note – the exercise pulls up and away from round-shoulderedness.
Complete four circles slowly.

15   16

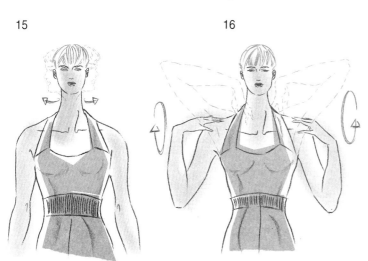

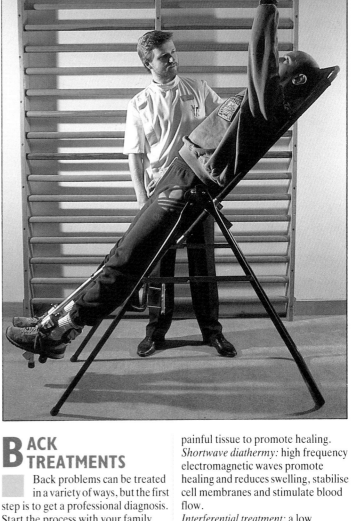

BACK TREATMENTS

Back problems can be treated in a variety of ways, but the first step is to get a professional diagnosis. Start the process with your family doctor, who may be able to refer you to an appropriate specialist or therapist. If you wish to consult a practitioner other than your doctor, consider the following:

● If your pain has not eased within 14 days but is bearable, consult a fully qualified orthopaedic physician, osteopath, chiropractor or physiotherapist.

● For recurring periods of back and neck pain see a physiotherapist, chiropractor, osteopath or an orthopaedic physician.

● For relentless chronic back pain see an orthopaedic specialist, a homoeopath, an acupuncturist, osteopath or chiropractor. Some of these therapies can be combined.

● If you suspect your back pain may be caused by an allergy, ask your doctor for an allergy test. (See ALLERGIES.)

● Electronic equipment can give relief and help promote healing.
Ultrasound: treats soft tissue injuries such as damage to muscle, ligament and tendon. High frequency soundwaves are focused directly on

painful tissue to promote healing.
Shortwave diathermy: high frequency electromagnetic waves promote healing and reduces swelling, stabilise cell membranes and stimulate blood flow.
Interferential treatment: a low frequency interference wave is produced where two medium frequency alternating currents coincide. This is used to reduce inflammation in joints and muscles.
Transcutaneous nerve stimulation: helps relieve severe pain. An electrical current passes between two surface electrodes on painful areas. Can be worn during the day.
Traction: gently pulls spinal joints apart enabling muscles to relax fully and reduce pressure on discs. If pain is experienced as traction is being put on and increased, ask the therapist to stop and don't continue.

● Injections are an effective way of treating a specific trouble spot.
Muscular injections: local injections of small doses of corticosteroid and local anaesthetic should be combined with stretching exercises to help muscles relax.
Ligament injections: ligament injuries are slow to heal. Small amounts of steroid with local anaesthetic can be injected along the length of the ligament. You will need to rest for at least ten days afterwards.

BAD BREATH

Poor oral health and poor digestion are the two main causes of unpleasant breath. A lack of digestive enzymes may cause the smell of incompletely digested food to come up through the oesophagus, the throat and finally through the mouth. Most digestion-related bad breath is caused by caffeine, refined sugar, white flour and cow's milk.

Throat infections, dirty dentures, alcohol, tobacco and mouth ulcers also cause bad breath.

Cleaning teeth regularly, maintaining healthy gums (plenty of vitamin C), and gently brushing the tongue are the best preventative measures.

Ask your dentist to recommend a hygienist who will advise you on a thorough oral hygiene routine.

Strong food smells such as GARLIC can be dispelled by chewing parsley. Gargle regularly with rosewater or lavender water.

BATHING

The therapeutic benefits of bathing have been acclaimed by civilisations throughout history. A good bath not only washes away the day's grime, but calms and relaxes, so it's worth celebrating…

To soak in an aromatic bath, sprinkle about six drops of an ESSENTIAL OIL on the surface of the water and stir to disperse the oil just before getting in. If skin is sensitive or the bath is for a baby or young child, dilute the oil in a light vegetable or sunflower oil, or in three tablespoons of full-fat milk.

Choose an oil to suit your mood: peppermint for fatigue; bergamot to cheer and uplift, and for its deodorant and antiseptic properties; invigorating rosemary for a morning bath before work; heady jasmine for a party. Rose, orange flower and clary sage are said to be aphrodisiacs, so they're wonderful for sharing a bath with someone special.

A spoonful of honey added to the bathwater is said to aid sleep. To soften skin and soothe aching muscles, add a cupful of cider vinegar and soak for 20 minutes. A good bath oil can be made by mixing a cupful of light vegetable oil with a teaspoonful of herbal shampoo. Itchy skin can be soothed by placing four camomile tea bags in the bath water.

After bathing give yourself a friction rub – stand in the bath or shower with the cold water running and use a loofah or bath brush to scrub your skin all over. Rub handfuls of sea salt – an excellent exfoliant – over your body and shower off. This leaves the skin tingling and glowing.

Afterwards gently massage your body with a natural oil such as almond, sesame or olive.

An Epsom salts bath is ideal during the early stages of a cold, or after exposure to damp, cold weather. (But not recommended for the very young, the elderly, or those with high blood pressure.) Fill a bath with enough water to cover your shoulders, as hot as you can comfortably bear it. Dissolve two handfuls of unpurified Epsom salts in the water.

Place a cold COMPRESS on your forehead and soak for no more than 20 minutes. Get out of the bath carefully, wrap yourself in a sheet and get into a warmed bed to encourage perspiration.

For back problems, genital and rectal complaints, you could try the old-fashioned sitz bath: use two large bowls, fill one with hot water, the other with cold. Place your feet in the cold and sit in the hot water for approximately three minutes. Switch round for one minute, then repeat the routine three times.

BEAUTY

Beauty is not just skin deep; it comes from an inner radiance that has little to do with perfect features, cosmetics or youth. Some of the world's plainest and oldest people are considered beautiful. Their beauty comes from the vitality of good health and a genuine love of themselves and the world around them. They have achieved a harmonious balance between the four main strands of human life – the physical, the mental, the emotional and the spiritual. Neglect any of these elements and beauty quickly fades – beauty is not merely what you look like, it is what you are, and what you are manifests itself in your lifestyle – the way you choose to lead your life. You can be as beautiful as you want to be!

● You can't be beautiful if you have a poor diet and a sedentary lifestyle. Skin will not be clear, eyes will not sparkle and hair will not shine. A balanced DIET – plenty of vegetables and fruit, and no junk foods – combined with regular EXERCISE will bring the sparkle back to your looks and boost energy.

● If you cannot express your

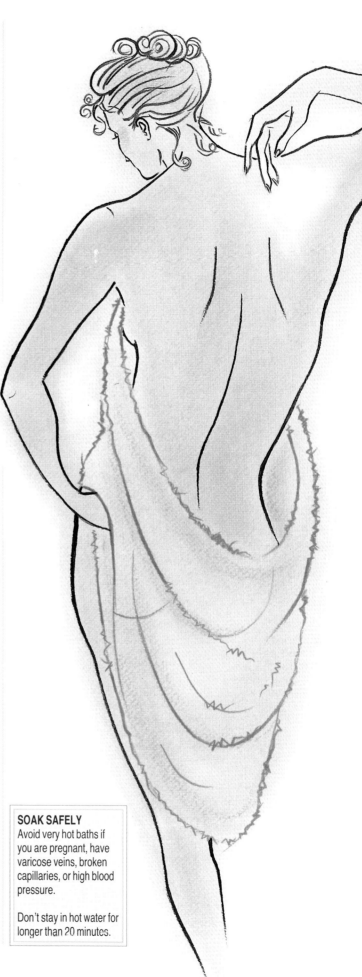

SOAK SAFELY

Avoid very hot baths if you are pregnant, have varicose veins, broken capillaries, or high blood pressure.

Don't stay in hot water for longer than 20 minutes.

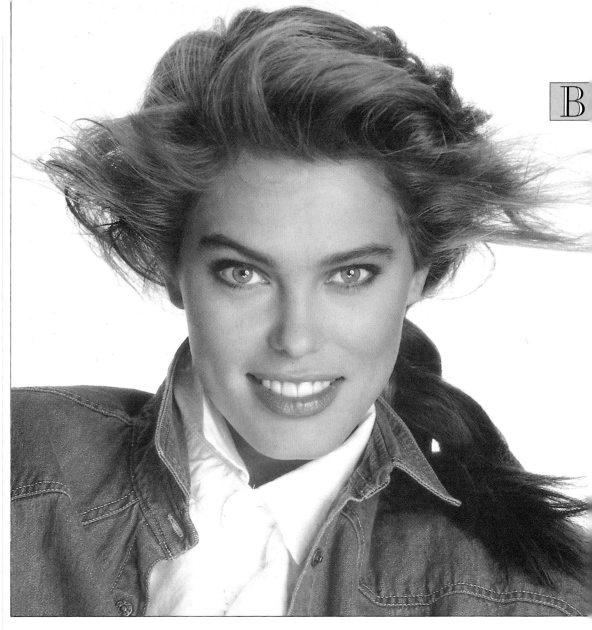

emotions, the anger, anxiety and despair will reveal themselves in the contorted muscles of your face and posture. Acknowledging and expressing your feelings is part of developing a strong sense of self – not how others would like you to be, but as you *really* are. Self-love promotes self-confidence and, as well as nurturing an inner beauty, is a prerequisite for loving others. (See EMOTION, COUNSELLING.)

● A lively curiosity for the world around you and a keen thirst for knowledge keeps mental faculties alert. Enthusiasm for interests outside work and home broadens the mind, makes you a stimulating and interesting person to be with.

● Spirituality does not necessarily mean going to church every Sunday. It is a reverential, sublime expression of how we relate to something greater than ourselves.

For some this is God in the Christian sense, for others it is Nature, Allah, the Goddess, or some concept of The Good. In an outward sense we may touch upon our spirituality through ritual, prayer, chanting, meditation and discipline of the body – resolving stress and nourishing our inner selves.

BIOFEEDBACK

This is a sophisticated method for learning to control biological responses, such as blood pressure, muscle tension and heart rate, through monitored relaxation. Electrical instruments measure physiological responses and make them apparent to the patient, who then tries to alter and control them without the aid of the monitoring devices.

In a typical treatment, sensors are attached to your forehead to measure muscle tension, and you are told to focus on relaxing images – such as lying on the beach listening to the waves. When you have concentrated long enough on that image the muscles in your forehead should relax. The change will be monitored by the meter in front of you. After several training sessions, you will be able to create a relaxed bodily state within minutes.

Biofeedback helps patients to relax muscles or adjust blood flow, so is ideal for those suffering from stress-related conditions such as headaches, eczema and high blood pressure.

BIORHYTHMS

Biorhythms are believed to be set in motion by the trauma of birth. The shock of leaving the safe, warm confines of the womb sets off a series of three cycles which continue to reoccur at regular intervals throughout life.

The physical cycle lasts 23 days, the emotional cycle 28 days and the intellectual cycle 33 days. Each cycle charted on a graph forms a wave pattern. A critical period of the month is reached when the cycles cross each other on one particular day. During these critical periods you are believed to be more prone to accidents and illness. Knowledge of your biorhythms can help you avoid emotional confrontations, major decisions, long journeys etc, on days when you are least likely to cope easily. There are biorhythms agencies who will provide a computer print-out for a six to 12-month period once they have your birthdate. It is presented as a graph, so you can see at a glance critical days and periods of harmony. Biorhythmic calculators are also available.

Biorhythms can give people a feeling that they are in control of certain areas of their life and able to avoid potentially stressful situations.

BLOOD PRESSURE

The pressure of blood in the circulatory system is a key indicator of the state of health of your heart, veins and arteries.

Blood pressure fluctuates during the day, depending on what you are doing; it rises with physical exertion and falls at rest. When measured by a sphygmomanometer normal blood pressure is about 120mm of mercury (mm Hy) systolic pressure (when heart contracts) and 80mm Hy diastolic pressure (when the heart relaxes). These measurements are often written as 120/80 – a normal reading, depending on age.

The sphygmomanometer is a familiar piece of equipment in any doctor's surgery. It consists of a pneumatic armlet connected by a rubber tube to an air pressure pump and gauge. When the armlet is wrapped around the upper arm the pressure obliterates the pulse and the level of the mercury in the gauge indicates the systolic blood pressure.

When blood pressure is consistently high or abnormally low, serious problems can occur. Women taking the contraceptive pill should have their blood pressure checked regularly. (See HYPERTENSION-high blood pressure, HYPOTENSION-low blood pressure, HEALTH CHECKS.)

BODY ODOUR

Sweat is part of your body's cooling mechanism, and is produced by the eccrine and apocrine glands. It contains mineral salts, protein and certain fatty substances. It doesn't smell; the odour is caused by bacteria on the skin attracted to the sweat.

The most effective way to combat body odour is to wash every day. If you are particularly prone to body odour, try to shower as frequently as you can, first hot to encourage perspiration and then cold to close your skin pores.

When buying aerosol deodorants and anti-perspirants, think of the environment as well as your armpits. Some aerosols contain chlorofluorocarbons (CFCs) which can destroy the earth's protective ozone layer. (See GREEN.) Always check that you are buying a CFC-free brand, or buy a roll-on instead. Deodorants restrict the action of the bacteria of the skin, and anti-perspirants control odour by restricting perspiration. Some of these products contain aluminium and zinc salts that prevent sweat reaching the skin and may cause swelling and blockage of sweat ducts.

Some essential oils, such as rose and lavender, can help treat body odour: sprinkle no more than six drops of either in your bath water. Supplements of magnesium and zinc have been found to act as 'internal deodorants'.

For sweet reminders, place sachets of herbs and dried flowers among your clean underwear.

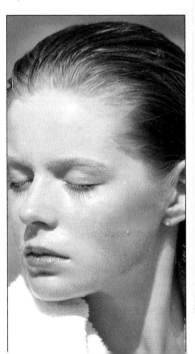

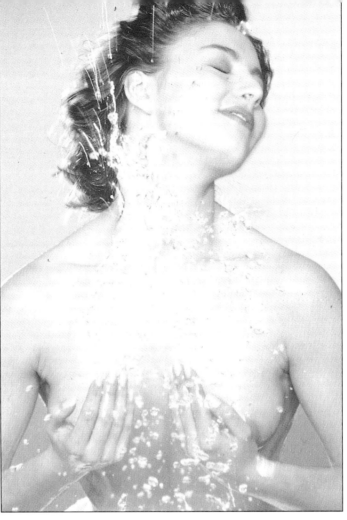

BREASTS

Posture, pregnancy, an increase in weight, the contraceptive pill, loss of weight, lack of firm support, the passing of time and genetic inheritance are all factors affecting the size, firmness and shape of breasts.

Excessive worry about breast shape and firmness can mask an overall insecurity or a general lack of confidence. Accepting and liking your breasts is a step towards liking and accepting yourself and boosting self-confidence. The popular obsession with breasts as an erogenous zone detracts from the real purpose of breasts – to nourish and comfort babies.

Breasts consist of fatty and glandular tissue. There is no muscle and each breast is supported by two ligaments called Cooper's ligaments. When these ligaments are stretched breasts start to droop. Short of COSMETIC SURGERY there is very little a woman can do to improve them, but there is a lot that can be done to maintain healthy breasts…

● *Exercise regularly* to keep chest and muscles strong for supporting your breasts. (As there are no muscles in the breasts exercise will not firm them, but stronger chest muscles will marginally improve uplift.) Swimming, especially breast stroke, is ideal. Passive exercising with FARADIC current equipment will also help, or try these exercises at home:

Place palms of your hands together in front of your chest, elbows out to the sides, and press together hard, feeling the chest muscles tighten as you do so. Hold for three seconds. Repeat 20 times, breathing deeply as you go.

Smile. Exaggerate into a grimace and feel the contraction of your neck muscles. Hold for five seconds. Repeat 20 times.

Good posture boosts self-image as well as breasts. Try slightly tilting the pelvis up and forward and tucking your bottom under. The straightening spine will lift the rib cage and breasts.

After a bath massage your breasts with your favourite moisturiser to keep skin supple and soft.

Support your breasts in a well fitting bra. Never exercise or take part in a sport without proper support. Jump up and down when trying on sports bras to make sure there is little bouncing and no pain.

BREAST EXAMINATION

Breast cancer is the commonest form of cancer in women living in Western countries. One in 12 women develop breast cancer and 35 women a day die from the disease in the UK. Yet many women live for years after having experienced breast cancer and treatment.

Very few lumps are actually malignant and breast changes can be caused by the contraceptive pill, pregnancy and menstruation.

Early diagnosis may give you greater options about treatment; it is possible to take some control over breast health and disease.

Regular self-examination of the breasts gives women a greater knowledge of how their breasts feel and of any changes. It is a very useful procedure, and it's well worth overcoming any anxiety you may have about it. It is best to be shown how to examine your breasts by an expert – workers at family planning clinics and Well Woman clinics will usually show you – and explanatory leaflets are freely available.

● If you are pre-menopausal, choose a day soon after your period ends to examine your breasts. This is important because breasts do change in size and density during your monthly cycle.

● Stand in front of a mirror and look carefully at your breasts.

● Notice any changes in size, puckering of the skin, bleeding or discharge from the nipples, changes in skin texture.

● Put your hands behind your head and swivel from side to side to see your breasts from different angles.

● Raise your arms to check breasts move together.

● Lean forward and examine each breast for any changes in outline or puckering.

● Get into a comfortable position lying down.

● Starting with the left breast and using the flat of your fingers (not the tips), press gently on the breast working in circular movements from the outside of the breast in towards the nipple. Feel for any lumps or changes. Breasts can be normally lumpy – get to know your lumps so that you can feel for unfamiliar ones.

● Check for lumps along the collar bone and in the armpit.

● If you think you have found an abnormal lump, check again the next day, and if it is still present consult your doctor.

● Report any unusual swelling in the upper arm or armpit.

BREAST MAMMOGRAPHY

Mammography is an X-ray examination of the breast to show internal structure. It can detect cancer at a very early stage, locating abnormalities too small to be felt in a normal breast examination.

Modern mammography exposes the breast to a tiny amount of radiation. The procedure is simple and painless. It is necessary to undress to the waist for the examination. During the X-ray your breasts will be slightly compressed to provide a better picture. This may be slightly uncomfortable but it lasts for only a few seconds. Breast cancer is rare in young women and mammography is normally used for women over 35 for diagnostic purposes.

By the 1990s all women between the ages of 50 and 64 should be automatically offered mammography by the NHS every three years. Women over 64 will be entitled to a mammogram on request. (See HEALTH CHECKS.)

A high proportion of mammograms show abnormality of some kind and women are required to have further mammograms or undergo further investigations.

BREATHING

Each time we breathe in we supply our cells with the life-giving oxygen they need. Each time we breathe out we are ridding our body of some of its wastes – particularly carbon dioxide.

Most of us don't know how to breathe correctly and use only half our breathing potential. As a result we not only miss out on its health-giving qualities but also fail to use it fully as an essential aid to beauty.

Correct breathing reduces the build up of toxins in the body's system which occurs when breathing is too shallow. It aids digestion by massaging the digestive organs. Increased oxygen revitalises the brain and nerve cells and stimulates the production of uplifting endorphins. Skin takes on a new radiance.

When you develop a good breathing technique thoughts become clearer and your entire body is energised. Here's how:
- Relax the stomach and solar plexus
- Breathe in through your nose using your whole chest and abdomen
- Put your hands on your stomach and check that it swells out. (When you inhale the muscles of the abdomen should draw the diaphragm down)
- Through your mouth breathe out all the air you have taken in.

Breathing can be used to reduce stress, depression and fatigue and in meditation it is the body's main tool for relaxation and entering deep mediative states. (See YOGA, RELAXATION.)

This deep breathing exercise is good for relieving tension, and can be done anywhere. Try it…
- Stand comfortably, with arms to the side
- Breathe slowly through your nose
- As you breathe in hunch up shoulders as high as you can, clench fists, stand on tiptoes, and tense your body harder and harder
- Sink back to your heels holding your breath
- Still holding breath loosen shoulders
- Exhale slowly through your nose as

BREATHING FACTS

Seven per cent of the oxygen we breathe in is used directly by the skin

Studies show that senility and vaguenessofthoughtinoldagecanbe causedbytoolittleoxygenbeingmade available to our cells through shallow breathing

We breathe on average 20 times a minute

Our lungs hold five litres of air when fully expanded, depending on height, age and sex

A man at rest breathes in about 3.75 litres of air per minute

you unclench your fists.
Repeat six times.

Breathing is also linked to our emotions. When we are excited breathing becomes shallower and faster, but fear and panic will have us gasping great lungfuls of air.

If you are in a situation in which you feel you have no control and are experiencing intense anger, sorrow or fear, try to concentrate on your breathing – taking deep, slow breaths calms the mind, reduces tension and also helps you to feel more in control of yourself and the situation.

Singing, MEDITATION and AUTOGENICS are effective ways of good for improving your breathing techniques.

BULIMIA NERVOSA

Bulimic sufferers starve themselves, then go on periodic binges where enormous quantities of food are consumed in a frenzy and always in secret.

Well-stocked cupboards and refrigerators are raided overnight. Raw meat and foods in their frozen state are often consumed in large quantities. The binge is followed by self-induced vomiting or by taking enormous doses of laxatives to maintain a normal body weight.

Bulimia nervosa is a particularly disturbing and destructive condition.

It can lead to stomach ruptures and severe intestinal disorders. Damage is caused to the colon, the oesophagus and throat. Long-term effects include hair loss, kidney failure and acute depression. The teeth decay and the skin around the eyes becomes bloated.

Most bulimics are prone to being overweight, but by their strange habits manage to maintain a normal weight.

They are often able to camouflage their condition far more satisfactorily than anorexics, as they are not as emaciated and in a social situation usually appear to be eating normally. But the root causes of bulimia nervosa are very similar to those of anorexia nervosa.

Appropriate treatment includes psychotherapy – often with the sufferer's family – and nutritional counselling. Many hospitals now offer out-patient consultation for bulimics.

BUTTOCKS

These two cushions of fat and muscle are often the first parts of the body to go flabby because of too much time spent sitting at a desk, in the car, or in bed. Do remember that Youth need not have a monopoly on tight, sleek buttocks.
- A simple daily exercise such as clenching the buttocks so tight they hurt, holding for ten seconds, then relaxing and repeating, is an excellent firmer that need only take a few minutes.
- Or try sitting on the floor, knees up to the chin, hands clasped around knees, and rock backwards as far as you can so that shoulders are on the floor and seat is in the air. Rock forwards to sitting position again. Repeat ten times.
- The buttocks seem to acquire extra weight easily, so watch diet – cut out sugar and refined foods. Walk as much as you can, and try the following exercise.
- Stand erect, arms by side. Tighten buttocks as hard as you can, tuck base of spine underneath hard, and pull abdominal muscles in and up towards ribs and spine.

Relax buttocks and tilt base of spine out as much as you can.

Repeat standing and then on all fours.
- Skin in this area can be rough and spotty – mainly because of sitting, sluggish circulation and tight underwear. So regular EXFOLIATION is a must, and always moisturise thoroughly after a bath.
- The buttocks are an area of the body that gets particularly tense, especially beneath the small of the back. Get a friend to massage out those knots of tension with a creamy massage lotion, rather than an oil.

Feels good!

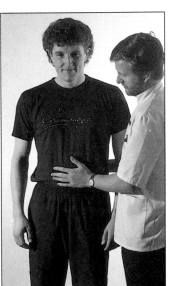
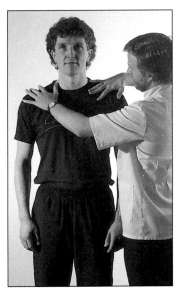

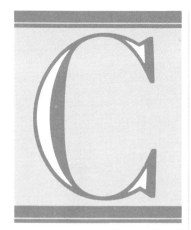

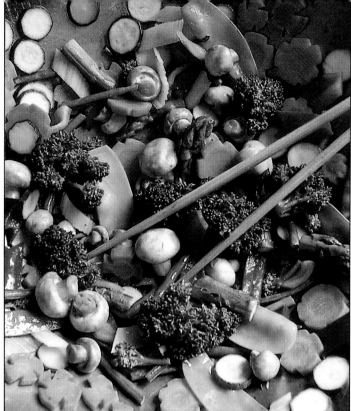

CALORIES

Food intake is expressed in units of potential energy called calories. A kilocalorie (kcal) is the amount of energy required to raise one kilogram of water one degree centigrade in temperature. When we refer to calories in our diet, it is really kilocalories we are talking about.

A sedentary worker needs approximately 1,800 kcals a day. A more active person may need between 2,500 and 3,000 kcals. A certain amount of these calories will be used by the body to maintain all the normal body processes, and this is called the basal metabolic rate. The rest is used up by movement of the body or stored as fat.

The calorie content in food varies. Protein and carbohydrate foods supply four calories per gram while fat provides approximately 9 calories per gram. The amount of calories used varies according to the type of activity; an hour's brisk walking uses 200 calories. while half an hour of energetic cycling will use up 250 calories. The clear rule is – if you eat less than you burn, you get thinner. (See SLIMMING, DIET, OVERWEIGHT.)

CAMOUFLAGE

Unsightly facial scars, blemishes, moles and birthmarks can be camouflaged by the skilful use of waterproof make-up. It is advisable to have lessons with a specially trained beauty therapist who will select the correct colours for your skin and show you how to blend and apply make-up with a brush or fingertips. Camouflage can be very effective and not expensive. It can also be used to cover varicose veins.

CARBOHYDRATES

Carbohydrates are one of the three main building blocks of life – the others are proteins and fats. Used mainly as a source of energy, carbohydrates are composed of carbon, hydrogen and oxygen and are found in all living cells.

Simple carbohydrates are digested quickly, while complex carbohydrates are digested slowly, making them a better source for stamina and continued energy.

Fruit juices, white and brown sugar, honey and milk products are all simple carbohydrates.

Grains, lentils, beans, potatoes, wholemeal pasta and brown rice are complex carbohydrates.

Each gram of carbohydrate provides the body with a little over four kcals of energy.

Most of the carbohydrates in a typical Western diet, such as sugars and syrups, have been so refined as to give practically no food value at all. They quickly raise the level of cholesterol and other blood fats, setting the consumer on the road to heart disease, as well as various blood sugar disorders.

The cause of diabetes mellitus is the inability of the body to assimilate and process carbohydrates.

Unrefined carbohydrates, such as whole grains, fresh fruit and vegetables, metabolise more slowly, releasing glucose into the bloodstream at a rate which will maintain energy levels, health, and brain function. (The brain uses 25 per cent of all glucose in your body.)

Indigestible forms of carbohydrate called FIBRE play a crucial role in the digestive system. They slow down absorption of sugars, preventing high levels of sugar in the bloodstream, speed the passage of digested food through the intestines, prevent gall stones and reduce cholesterol levels. (See DIET.)

CARDIOVASCULAR EXERCISE

Any activity which gets the heart and lungs working harder can be termed cardiovascular exercise. No fitness programme is complete without a cardiovascular endurance exercise characterised by repeatedly and vigorously moving the major muscles of the body for an extended period of time. Fit heart and lungs increase the body's ability to take in, pump and utilise its oxygenated blood. The pay-off is more energy, less stress, sound, deep sleep and a feeling that you're on top of the world!

Choose an aerobic activity such as swimming, jogging or cycling and work out regularly, starting gently at first and slowly building up as your heart and lungs become stronger. (See AEROBICS, EXERCISE.) Skipping is the simplest form to do at home.

CELLULITE

Those lumps and bumps that won't go away are fat tissue telling you something about your diet, habits and sedentary lifestyle. Affecting only women, cellulite consists of areas of fat with excess fluid, restricts blood-carrying capillaries and seeps between the cells making skin look puffy.

Over the years, fibrils of COLLAGEN surround the fat cells, restricting capillaries and blood supply. Wastes accumulate and nutrients vital for the cells' healthy growth are blocked. Circulation of blood and lymph (essential for the drainage and removal of toxins in the body) becomes sluggish. When pinched, the skin dimples and looks like orange peel. Cellulite affects mainly the thighs, upper arms, abdomen and buttocks, and you don't have to be fat to have it. (See LYMPHATIC SYSTEM.)

To banish cellulite and prevent it ever paying a return visit you need to launch a concerted campaign on your body. This means major lifestyle changes and some extra pampering.

FIRST, REVAMP YOUR DIET

Avoid foods containing unnecessary preservatives and additives, which encourage build-up of toxic waste and excess fluid. Eat plenty of fresh fruit and vegetables. Cut down on salt – another fluid retainer. Eat plenty of potassium-rich foods such as potatoes, spinach, bananas, beans and fruit juices.

Fresh pineapple and grapes are thought to break down body fats. Water melon contains a natural diuretic which flushes out excess fluids from the body. Eat plenty of celery, too, and drink lots and lots of water. Nettle and fennel teas are also recommended.

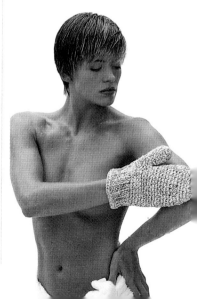

QUIT SMOKING

Cigarettes encourage the build-up of cellulite by breaking down collagen – essential for maintaining the skin's elasticity and firmness. Nicotine impairs the absorption of vitamins essential for the skin's health, such as vitamins C and B, and carbon monoxide restricts capillaries that feed blood to the tissues, so circulation becomes sluggish.

GET EXERCISING

Boost circulation, increase the oxygen in your blood and start eliminating waste efficiently! Any AEROBIC activity will be especially beneficial. To beat cellulite, an exercise programme should be combined with regular massage.

THE MASSAGE MESSAGE

Knotted muscles caused by a period of stress can cause toxic build-up and restrict lymphatic drainage. Massage relaxes the muscles and stimulates the circulation.

Treat yourself to a course of aromatherapy massage. One or a combination of several of the following essential oils are likely to be used – geranium, rosemary, black pepper, fennel and juniper. Combined with a specialised massage to drain and stimulate the lymphatic system, the oils are very effective. HYDROTHERAPY and ROLFING are also effective therapies for combating cellulite.

Brushing the skin with a sisal mitt or bristle brush before a shower or bath increases circulation. Massage tools with rubber nodules or rollers help soften collagen fibres. These can be used with body-contouring agents such as seaweed, vitamin E and plant extracts including ivy, horse-chestnut and butcher's broom.

Various treatments for cellulite are available at beauty salons and health resorts, where a qualified beauty therapist will be able to give you detailed advice.

CHIROPRACTIC

The word chiropractic comes from the Greek meaning 'treatment by manipulation'. American healer David Daniel Palmer discovered that by manipulating the spine he could treat other areas of the body. Convinced that the basis of disease was in the spine, he developed the theory that displaced vertebrae (the 27 bones forming the spine) restrict the spinal

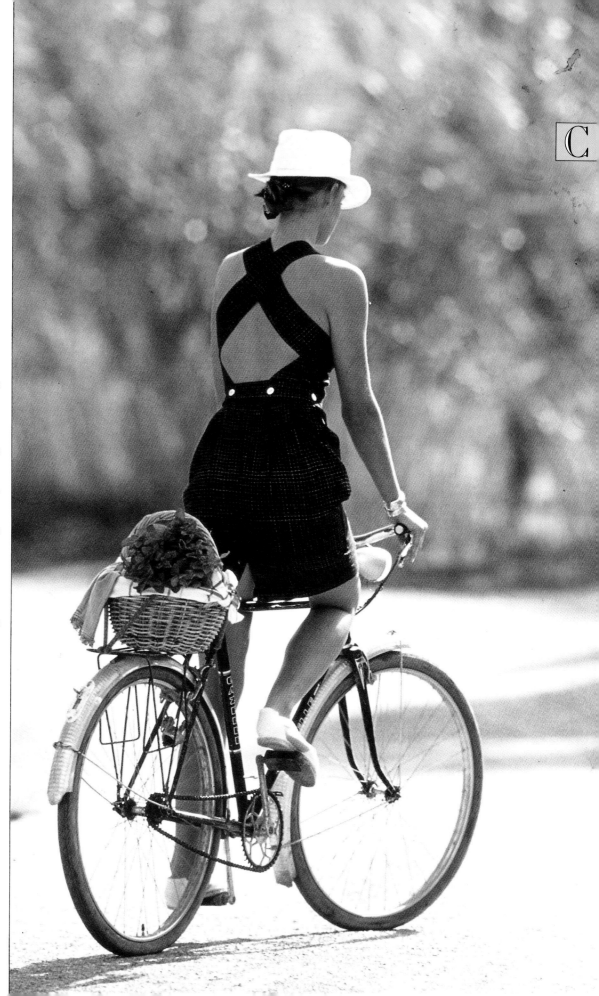

C

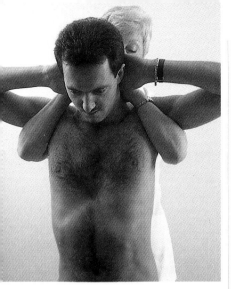

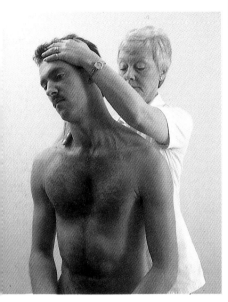

nerves and interfere with the body's nervous energy flow.

The treatment is closely allied to OSTEOPATHY. Both use manipulative techniques for musculoskeletal disorders, have a HOLISTIC approach to health and are concerned with preventative care. A chiropractor will use direct thrust against the joints or muscles and places great reliance on X-rays in the diagnosis. The emphasis is on adjusting the strains on specific joints using manual pressure. Soft tissue techniques may also be used – the ligaments and muscles are massaged to alleviate muscular pain and prepare a joint for manipulation. Sometimes you will hear the joints crack during treatment. Don't be alarmed! It's the sound of bubbles of nitrogen inside the joint cavities forming and dispersing as the joint is manipulated.

General joint problems, neuralgia, lumbago, strains, slipped discs and generalised back pain all respond well to chiropractic treatment. (See BACKS, BACK TREATMENT.)

CIRCULATION

Blood circulates around the body in a system of tubes or blood vessels of various sizes, arranged in two separate but interconnected circuits. The smaller circuit carries blood between the heart and lungs, and the larger takes blood around the rest of the body. In the lungs, oxygen is absorbed into the blood where, bright red and oxygenated, it flows to the heart via the pulmonary veins.

From the heart the blood is pumped through the arteries to make its circuit of the body, removing waste from the kidneys, taking up foodstuffs from the stomach and intestines to be processed by the liver, and delivering oxygen to the muscles and organs. It is then pumped back to the heart via a complex network of veins. Finally the blood, now duskier and deoxygenated is pumped into the lungs via the pulmonary arteries, to give up its waste carbon dioxide and pick up oxygen again.

A sluggish circulation is not only reflected in a dull complexion. It can affect muscles – cramp is a common sign of poor circulation, as are cold feet and hands and lethargy. For dynamic health and beauty, efficient circulation is essential.

To check your circulation is in good working order, press the tip of your big toe firmly against a hard surface for a few seconds and watch how long it takes to flush pink again after you let go. If you have to wait more than two seconds your blood isn't shifting as fast as it should.

To get circulation moving again take up an AEROBIC activity such as jogging, walking, swimming or cycling to get the heart and lungs working more efficiently. The signs of boosted circulation are immediate – notice the flushed cheeks and rise in body heat.

CIRCULATION FACTS

There are five litres of blood circulating in the body at any one time, holding one litre of oxygen – enough to keep a man alive for four minutes at rest, and less than a minute during exercise

Blood is pumped at a rate of five litres every minute. This can be increased to five litres every ten seconds

In an average lifetime, enough blood is circulated around the body to fill the Albert Hall

---

COLLAGEN

Beneath the surface of your skin lies a network of fibres which look like the weaving of a fine cloth. They are made up of a protein called collagen. Its water-holding ability gives the skin its smoothness and elasticity. Time, genetic factors, smoking, poor diet, pollution and lack of exercise cause the collagen fibres to harden, shift position and lose their water-retaining properties. The skin then starts to lose elasticity and firmness. Habitual facial expressions begin to inscribe themselves on your face, and WRINKLES form.

COLOUR

Imagine what it would be like to live in a room painted black. A depressing thought? The power of colour to affect mood was recognised thousands of years ago by both the Egyptians and Greeks. They decorated their temples with brilliant colours to uplift and promote a feeling of physical well-being.

Colour surrounds us. But do you make the most of it? Colour can lift us out of depression, heal, sedate, invigorate and boost our looks.

Colour therapy is believed to work well on stress-related conditions such as headaches, depression, irregular menstruation and back pain. Research shows that blue light lowers high blood pressure while red light raises it. Colour therapy has been used as emergency treatment for asthma – a blue light relaxes muscles and brings immediate relief.

Colour therapy is relatively new to this country and is usually applied via a Colour-Form-Rhythm-Beamer. The colour is beamed through a lens-like window in rhythmic waves, its intensity varying according to the amount of exposure required. Treatment lasts about 20 minutes and should be carried out at least three times a week until symptoms ease.

Colour also enhances your looks and life. Wearing the right colour can make you look younger, healthier, full of vitality and confidence.

Colour consultancy is an increasingly popular way to make the most of your own colouring through the right choice of colours to wear. A consultant will note your hair, skin and eye colour and decide which one of the four seasons you belong to – spring, summer, autumn or winter. For instance, winter includes most

olive-skinned people, blacks and Asians, as well as those with sallow skin. The hair is medium to dark brown or black, or grey. Winter eyes can be black-brown, red-brown, green-blue or hazel. If you're winter, you'll look good in bold, blue-based colours such as pine green, burgundy, fuchsia and dark navy.

The colour consultant will give you a chart of the colours you can mix and match depending on the season you are. Using your chart you will find yourself spending less time and energy shopping. You'll have more confidence and will know what to look for. And if you really hate clothes shopping, you can always give

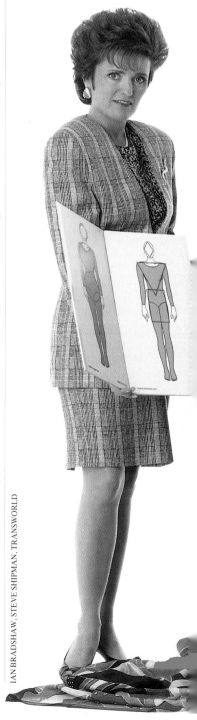

IAN BRADSHAW, STEVE SHIPMAN, TRANSWORLD

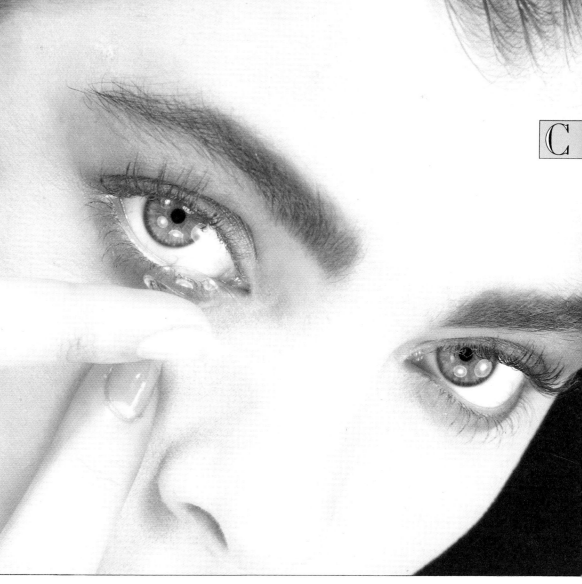

the chart to a friend to guide them straight to the right spot on the rack.

COMPRESSES

Hot compresses have been used for centuries to encourage the dilation of blood vessels, and should be applied to stiff, sore muscles. Take a large flannel and wring out in hot, not boiling, water, fold and cover the painful area. Leave the compress in

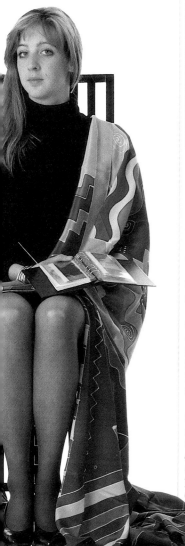

place until it has cooled.

A cold compress is excellent for subduing inflammation, such as that caused by a bruised knee or sore throat. Wring flannel out in cold water, bind in place with a bandage and leave for several hours or overnight.

The bandage should never be bound too tight, as circulation should not be at all impaired.

Alternate hot and cold compresses are suitable for any stiff or painful condition. Place the hot compress on the skin first for three minutes, followed by the cold for one minute. Repeat for 20 minutes, making fresh compresses when necessary.

For dry or flaky skin and to reduce swelling of a pulled muscle, try a comfrey compress. . .
● Put a handful of comfrey leaves in a cup of hot water.
● When cool, strain and place the wet leaves on muslin or gauze.
● Place on affected area. Leave for 15 minutes.

CONTACT LENSES

The basic theory of contact lenses appears in the 16th-century notes of Leonardo da Vinci. Today's contact lens is a tiny, paper-thin saucer of transparent plastic material shaped to fit over the cornea.

There are three main types of contact lenses – hard, soft and oxygen permeable. The micro corneal or hard contact lens lasts for many years and daily care is simple. They are less easy to get used to than soft lenses but carry far fewer risks of eye infection – unless you lick them instead of using the correct solution! Saliva contains bacteria.

The latest oxygen-permeable lenses are made from material which allows the direct passage of oxygen to the cornea. This means you can alternate between contact lenses and spectacles without the transient problem of spectacle blur.

Soft or hydrophilic lenses are larger than hard lenses and are made from a jelly-like material which absorbs water. When fully hydrated in a saline mixture they are completely soft and pliable. It is vital not to skimp on the sterilising procedures advised by manufacturers otherwise corneal infections can occur, some of which may cause blindness. Do not use home-made saline solutions for cleaning.

Soft lenses fall into two categories – Daily Wear lenses, worn during normal waking hours, and Extended Wear lenses, which may be worn day and night continuously and need only be removed about once a month.

Extended Wear lenses involve detailed consultation with the optician before fitting, carry the highest risk of infection and need to be handled delicately.

Hard micro corneal lenses are relatively inexpensive compared with soft lenses and in the long term often work out cheaper than spectacles.

A new alternative is the disposable soft lens. These are designed to be worn day and night for a week, then thrown away. They eliminate the need for daily cleansing and reduce the risk of infection. However, they are not available for people who are long-sighted.

Some contact lenses also come in a variety of colours, to match your wardrobe.

If you always feel like giving your eyes a rub when taking your contact lenses out, it could indicate that you are over-wearing them and not enough oxygen is reaching your eyes. Consult your optician – if the problem is not dealt with immediately, extra blood vessels will grow into the eye to compensate, thus impairing vision.

Exercise and sport should not stop you wearing contact lenses. Swimmers should wear hard or soft lenses with goggles (this applies to all water sports). Squash players should use proper eye protection whether they wear lenses or not, to avoid serious damage from ball or opponent's racket.

Contact lenses give freedom to skiers – it's not true that lenses freeze in your eyes while skiing.

Soft lenses are less easily dislodged than hard lenses, so are usually prescribed for boxing, rugby, soccer, diving and underwater swimming.

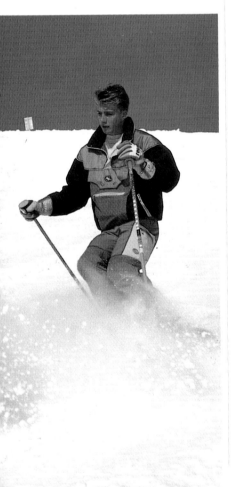

CONTRACEPTION

No contraceptive is 100 per cent safe, without unwanted side-effects and effortless for both partners.

Choice of contraception depends very much on to what extent pregnancy is unwanted, how long you wish to avoid pregnancy, whether or not both you and your partner are faithful, or whether you have several partners, and how much your sexual activities expose you to HIV, the Aids virus. Female and male sterilisation are the most effective ways to prevent conception, but may be considered too drastic by most people.

If you fail to use your chosen form of contraception, the morning-after pill for women can be taken – provided you consult your doctor or family planning clinic without delay. Two special doses of this pill are given up to 72 hours after sex. It is 96 to 99 per cent effective with correct and careful use.

The chart at the back of this book summarises the pros and cons of the most common forms of contraception.

COSMETIC SURGERY

More and more men and women are turning to the surgeon's scalpel to smooth out wrinkles, reshape noses, lift cheek-bones, breasts, necks, stomachs and chins. It's a costly business and there are the usual risks associated with operations and anaesthetics.

Cosmetic surgery will not solve all your problems and to benefit fully you need to have a healthy lifestyle (see BEAUTY) and be aware that a face-lift on its own will not bring happiness, though it may give you more confidence.

The first step is to find a good surgeon. Go via your GP explaining what you want and asking to be referred to a qualified plastic surgeon. If your doctor is dismissive you are within your rights to see another. The doctor will then obtain a list of qualified plastic surgeons from the College of Plastic Surgeons, part of the Royal College of Surgeons in London. It is inadvisable to make a direct approach to private clinics advertised in the popular press.

Collagen injections are a cheaper and less drastic form of cosmetic treatment, although the results are never long-lasting. Collagen can be

GUIDE TO MOST POPULAR COSMETIC OPERATIONS
(Prices are approximate)

Conventional face lift – skin only
Cost: £1,800–£2,300
Time: 3½ hrs
Possible side effects: temporary numbness, swelling, nerve injury

SMAS face lift – muscles lifted too
Cost: £2,500+
Time: 4–4½ hrs
Possible side effects: as for face lift but increased chances of bad bruising, swelling, nerve injury

Malar augmentation (cheekbone)
Cost: £1,500
Time: 1½ hrs
Possible side effects: risk of infection, displacement of implant, swelling

Blepharoplasty (eyelid surgery)
Cost: £950
Time: 2 hrs
Possible side effects: scars, undercorrection or over-correction (giving wide-eyed look), bruising

Brow lift
Cost: £1,500
Time: 1½ hrs
Possible side effects: prolonged numbness, over-correction creating very surprised expression

Rhinoplasty (nose job)
Cost: £1,500–£1,900
Time: 1 hr
Possible side effects: swelling for up to three weeks, infection. If too much bone is removed, there will be excessive scar replacement

Breast augmentation
Cost: £1,600
Time: 1 hr
Possible side effects: hardening of breast around implant

Breast reduction
Cost: £1,800–£2,300
Time: 1 hr
Possible side effects: loss of sensitivity in nipples, inability to breastfeed, bleeding and bad scarring.

Mastoplexy (breast uplift), can be combined with either of the above
Cost: £1,800
Time: 1½ hrs
Possible side effects: bad scarring, loss of sensitivity in the nipples

Body suction – fat is sucked out of thighs and abdomen
Cost: £1,500–£1,800
Time: 20–40 mins
Possible side effects: won't correct very ridged and dimply skin, a danger of over or undercorrection

used to get rid of wrinkles by filling out the skin from inside using a very fine needle.

Effects are temporary, lasting from six months to two years. You should have an allergy test first. Shrinking lips can also be plumped out with collagen injections.

A new development called fat autografting involves injecting deposits of fat from the thigh or tummy into the lips.

COUNSELLING

A counsellor is trained in special skills to help people sort out their emotional problems. A good counsellor will use communication skills to encourage people to talk about what is worrying them and discuss the underlying reasons to find a way to resolve them. For some people the opportunity to talk about their innermost thoughts and feelings is such a relief that the therapeutic value of counselling is soon apparent.

Marriage guidance is the most common form of counselling in this country, and many people opt for 'crisis' counselling to help them through a difficult period of their lives, such as bereavement or divorce.

Most British people have a genuine reserve about expressing their feelings and hold a common misconception that only the unstable or inadequate go for counselling. Nothing is farther from the truth; pent up emotions and unresolved problems gnaw away at the foundations of good health and erode potentially happy relationships. Repressed anger can cause depression, jealousy dulls the appetite, fear strains the heart and feelings of inadequacy and insecurity block a positive and optimistic outlook on life.

A good friend is always a safe shoulder to cry on, but very often it helps to talk to someone who can see the problem more clearly from the outside and who won't take sides if the problem is a marital one.

Most emotional problems are related to childhood, and an experienced counsellor is able to make these type of connections. Once you have a counsellor, expect to visit him or her every week until you feel you have resolved your difficulties.

The choice of counsellor is important. Always remember that you are the consumer – you choose your counsellor, they don't choose you. You have to feel you are entrusting your emotional pain and hurt to someone you can trust and like. The best counsellors are often those who have been through therapy themselves and have developed an understanding of the problems from both sides.

When choosing a counsellor:
● Make sure he or she has a qualification which suits your needs. A counsellor should have a counselling qualification, or be a trained psychotherapist.

If your problem is a sexual one, check that he or she is a fully trained sex therapist.

Ask the British Association for Counselling (address on following page, please enclose an sae) to send you a list of approved local counsellors, or contact your local branch of Relate (formerly the Marriage Guidance Council) who deal with all kinds of emotional problems.
● Make sure you feel safe and comfortable in the counselling room.
● Ask yourself, 'Would I be able to cry in front of this person?'
● Interview the counsellor. Make sure s/he understands issues that are important to you – for instance, if you are a woman struggling for independence make sure the counsellor understands the issues involved.

CRAVINGS

Regular food cravings indicate blood sugar imbalance or a food allergy.

Most cravings revolve around certain foods. For instance you may want to eat a whole packet of biscuits instead of just one or two. It's rather like being mildly addicted – the craving is difficult to resist. Women often have cravings, particularly for chocolate, just before menstruation when blood sugar levels tend to drop. Go for foods rich in B vitamins instead such as liver and whole grains.

Cravings can also be the way your body tells you it needs the minerals and vitamins of a certain food. If you suddenly have a craving for spinach for example, it may be that you are lacking in iron.

Craving salty foods? You could have adrenal deficiency as a result of stress. Cheese? You could need more calcium and phosphorous.

If you find yourself eating lots of nuts, you are probably under stress. A craving for apples could mean your diet contains a lot of saturated fats. (See OVERWEIGHT.)

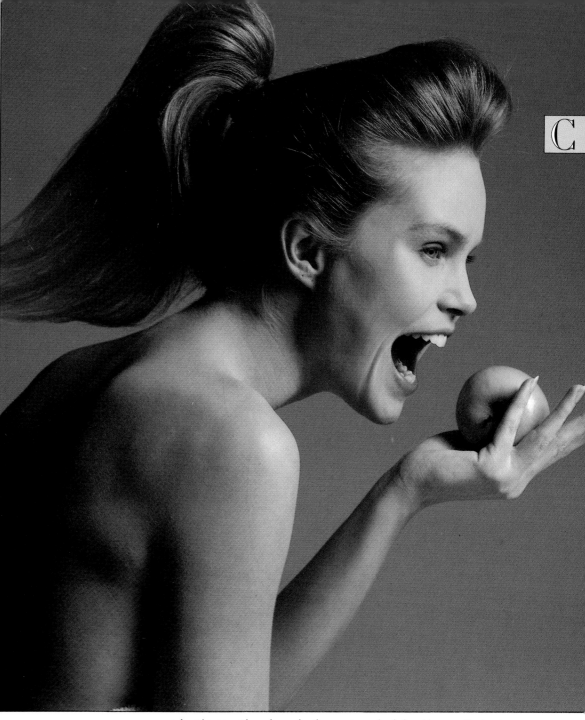

CYSTITIS

Approximately half the women in Britain suffer from this uncomfortable and painful condition. Cystitis is the inflammation of the bladder and is caused by a bacteria called Escherichia Coli which is found around the bowel opening. It is usually harmless but once inside the bladder it wreaks havoc. It is transferred from the bowel by sex, tampons, poor hygiene or by wearing tight trousers. Allergies, anxiety and depression can make the bladder susceptible to cystitis.

The symptoms are an intense burning sensation when urinating, and a very frequent desire to pass small quantities of urine. This may be accompanied by fever, cloudy or bloody urine and a dull ache in the lower back. In severe cases sufferers might experience high temperature and fits of shivering.

When suffering an acute attack, immediately implement the following plan of action:
● Drink a pint (575 ml) of water.
● Mix a drink of one teaspoon of bicarbonate of soda in a cup of warm water – take every three hours.
● Sip water frequently and drink parsley tea hourly – three teaspoons of fresh parsley/one teaspoon dried parsley infused in cup of hot water. (See HERBALISM.)
● Curl up with a hot water bottle on the abdomen, alternating with a cold wet towel, for five minutes only.
● Do not eat during attacks.
● If body temperature rises, apply a cold compress from armpit to groin and consult your doctor. (See COMPRESSES.)
● Always rinse gently and dry after you have passed water.
● Fluid intake should be a minimum of four litres per 24 hours during the acute phase.
● A doctor should be consulted and a urine sample will be sent to labs for culture and appropriate treatment.

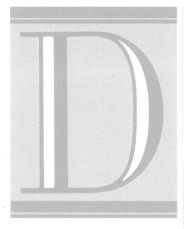

D

DANCE

Dancing is an exhilarating way to keep fit. It improves posture, flexibility, strength, endurance, breathing and agility, and can also enhance your social life! It has enormous therapeutic value – throughout the ages dance has been a creative form of expressing emotion, as well as a fulfilling way of celebrating and communicating with others.

There's a form of dance to suit everyone, regardless of age and sex, including ballet, jazz, ballroom, disco and folk. The benefits of dance and cardiovascular exercise are combined in aerobic dance. It keeps you moving constantly for 15 to 20 minutes and includes a wide range of movement from running on the spot to rumba and disco. For full benefit any aerobic activity should be done three to five times a week. (See AEROBIC, EXERCISE.)

Once initial self-consciousness has been overcome, along with the fear of stepping out on the wrong foot, dancing takes you over and becomes

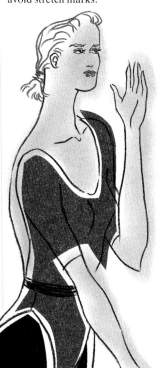

the perfect antidote to stress. The joy and ecstasy of pure motion and freedom overwhelm – caught up in the beat of the music, you forget yourself and your problems are pushed away.

Aerobic dance, ballet, vigorous jazz and modern dance are all top calorie burners, using up over 600 calories an hour. (See CALORIES) Belly dancing keeps the waist trim and burns up more calories than tennis. It was taught to Turkish brides to give them painless childbirth and avoid stretch marks.

DANDRUFF

A normal scalp is made up of between 30 to 40 layers of dead, dry skin cells. It takes approximately 28 days for the whole lot to slough off in clumps. Dandruff occurs when as many as 50 layers in larger clumps are lost over a shorter period.

Microbes, hormonal irregularities, infrequent shampooing, sunburned scalp and poor diet are all thought to trigger dandruff.

Oily scalps with dandruff (the hair will be greasy and the dandruff will feel oily) benefit from an anti-dandruff shampoo with zinc pyrithone. *Keep out of reach of children*. Apply a mild antiseptic such as diluted witch hazel afterwards. Milder shampoos should be used on drier scalps. A flaky scalp that feels tight is a sign of stress. While shampooing massage well until the scalp tingles. (See MASSAGE.)

Try using natural yoghurt as a conditioner. Wash hair, rinse, apply the yoghurt and rub in well. Leave for 15 minutes and rinse out. Wash again with just a drop of mild shampoo.

DEPRESSION

Almost everyone experiences depression – usually after a loss of some kind such as bereavement, divorce, redundancy.

What distinguishes the illness of depression from a normal fluctuation of mood is that it is deeper and more long-lasting. When you are suffering severe depression and not just a dose of the blues, you may hate yourself and everyone else, and speak slowly in a monotone. You may find it difficult to concentrate or make a simple decision. Sleep is restless, you often wake up much earlier than usual and can't get back to sleep. You feel frustrated, trapped and hopeless.

Twice as many women as men suffer from depression. Pregnancy, childbirth, menopause and the contraceptive pill can all trigger the condition.

Research in Britain and America shows that a wide variety of factors can cause depression:

● Deficiencies in diet such as calcium and magnesium, vitamin B9, vitamin B6 (pyridoxine), and the amino acids tryptophan and tyrosine.
● Low blood sugar (hypoglycaemia), countered by eating a diet rich in PROTEIN and free of refined CARBOHYDRATES and coffee.

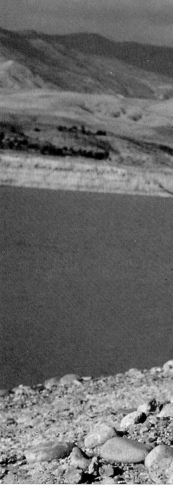

● Unexpressed anger – if turned inward this strong emotion sets off a depressive response to life. There are ways of expressing anger without hurting anyone. COUNSELLING and psychotherapy can help.
● Drinking more than four cups of coffee a day.
● Allergies to food and chemicals in the environment such as pesticides, herbicides etc.
● Winter – it is now known that a lack of sunlight can cause 'winter depression' or Seasonal Affected Disorder (SAD). Sufferers benefit from exposure to certain wavelengths of light.

Don't let your doctor give you a prescription for powerful medicines without proper discussion. Anti-depressants can help, but should only be used as a last resort. Make sure your doctor explains exactly what is being prescribed, what it's for and any side effects.

Check whether or not you should avoid eating certain foods while taking the drug. Avoid all cheese, meat and yeast extracts (Oxo, Bovril, Marmite), broad bean pods, pickled herrings, bananas, yoghurt, chocolate, canned figs, red wine and sherry if you are taking anti-depressants.

There are other ways to combat

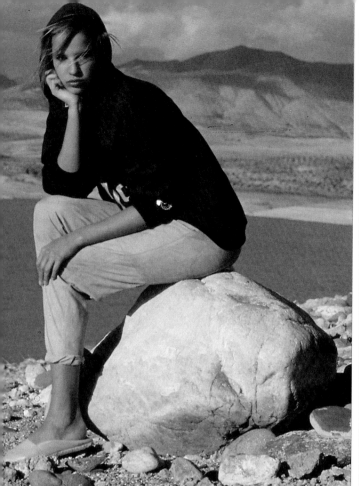

depression. Exercise has been shown to aid recovery, as the main problem is often overcoming one of the major symptoms of depression – lethargy. Regular exercise releases chemicals in the brain called endorphins which lift the spirits. A brisk 20 minute walk each day can work wonders.

Dietary supplements may be needed and herbal remedies such as hops, passiflora, valerian and lavender have proved helpful to some, as have homoeopathic remedies. The therapeutic value of massage combined with essential oils that uplift (geranium, melissa, rose) or sedate (camomile, ylang-ylang) can help shift the dark clouds that seem to engulf a depressed person.

The most effective approach to depression is psychotherapy. Encouraging the depressive to talk about their problems and enhancing self-awareness either in counselling or group therapy is the first step towards recovery. Although it is easy to lose patience with a depressed person, friends and relatives play an essential part in helping them overcome their misery through showing love and understanding. Telling a depressed person to 'pull yourself together', will only make matters worse.

D IET

You are what you eat. If your diet is inadequate, your body will find ways of letting you know sooner or later. Extra weight, spotty skin, lethargy, constipation, dental decay and heart disease can all indicate an unbalanced diet.

Healthy eating is not only governed by the kinds of food that you eat, but also by your lifestyle, which affects your eating habits. The body needs time to relax, digest and absorb food in addition to being provided with the appropriate amounts of energy and nutrients required for daily activities.

A good diet maintains health, promotes growth, provides energy, protects against disease, and helps you look good too!

Adopting a new food philosophy can be fun and is an exciting opportunity to try new tastes, dishes and cooking skills.

● Start by reducing intake of refined carbohydrates such as white flour and sugar. Daily sugar consumption shouldn't exceed 2oz (55g) a day; preferably cut it out altogether.

● Make sure at least 60 per cent of your diet contains fresh seasonal vegetables and fruit. Eat whole grain every day.

● Cut down on animal protein and replace with a variety of beans, peas, lentils and other pulses.

● Decrease your total fat intake. Choose lean meats, low fat dairy products and use low fat cooking methods. Drink no more than one pint of milk a day and less if you want to lose weight.

● Eat wholemeal bread, and wholegrain cereals in salads, or in soups and stews. They're delicious and beneficial.

● Judge your body's energy and nutritional requirements; eat to live, don't live to eat.

Your energy from food will decrease as you get older, eat slightly less and remain active to avoid an increase in weight.

● Eat nuts and dried fruits instead of sweets and chocolates.

● Drink at least two to four pints of water each day.

● Do not overcook fruit and vegetables – it causes loss of vitamins and minerals.

Either steam or use only a small amount of water and cook to just soften in order to retain as much goodness as possible.

Use the cooking water from vegetables in soups, gravies and sauces.

FOUR GOLDEN RULES FOR HEALTHY EATING

1 Cut down on fat, sugar and salt
2 Eat fibre-rich foods every day
3 Eat plenty of fresh fruit and vegetables
4 Get plenty of variety in what you eat

● Remember that most of the goodness of fruit and vegetables is found in the skin and immediately under it.

● Try to replace coffee and tea with decaffeinated products, herbal teas and fruit juices. (See CARBOHYDRATES, PROTEINS, FIBRE.)

REVITALISE YOUR EATING HABITS

The Champneys ten-day healthy eating plan overleaf can be used as a revitalising diet – ridding your body of toxins – and as an inspiration for changing unhealthy eating habits.

The eating plan provides all the protein, carbohydrates and fibre your body needs to maintain health and energy. Not only will it add some exciting new dishes to your kitchen repertoire, it will provide a wonderful way of treating yourself, family and friends. It shows that you can eat well and healthily without feeling deprived. And because it contains a lot of raw vegetables, you won't have to spend a lot of time preparing meals.

Do not follow the plan for more than ten days. If you are being treated for any illness, consult a doctor first. After the ten days of inspiration, you'll find it easier to keep to the four golden rules for healthy eating (above).

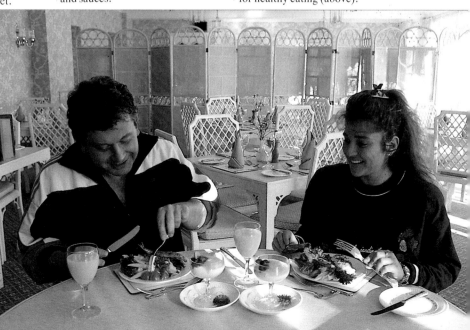

	Breakfast	Lunch	Evening
Day 1	Selection of favourite fruits and their juices or just mineral water		
Day 2	Large fruit salad and natural yoghurt	Mixed salad and sliced avocado Sprouted sunflower seeds Vegetable juice Fruit of choice	Gazpacho soup Bean and chickpea salad Fruit of choice
Day 3	Large fruit salad and natural yoghurt	Mixed salad Soused mackerel in strips and vegetable juice Fruit of choice	Gazpacho soup Mixed salad Sliced avocado Sprouted wheat
Day 4	Fruit salad Toast and tomatoes	Mixed salad Butter bean soup and bread Yoghurt and honey	Swedish trout Crisp new potatoes Baked apple with raspberries
Day 5	Fruit salad Muesli and milk/yoghurt	Mixed salad Stilton and herb pâté Jacket potato Fruit of choice	Turkey Helena Wholewheat tagliatelle Apricot and oat crumble
Day 6	Fruit salad Omelette and wholemeal bread	Chickpea salad Pitta bread Yoghurt and honey	Fish kebab and brown rice Cheese and crackers
Day 7	Fruit salad Muesli and milk/yoghurt	Sprouted salad Jacket potato Fruit of choice	Fillet of beef Crisp new potatoes Chestnut mousse
Day 8	Fruit salad Toast and tomatoes	Baked avocado with cheese sauce Wholemeal bread Yoghurt and honey	Halibut steaks au poivre Boiled new potatoes in skins Raspberry and mango flan
Day 9	Fruit salad Muesli and milk/yoghurt	Tuna fish coleslaw Jacket potato Sliced pineapple and mango	Calves liver with red wine Oaty potatoes Apricot and pistachio ice cream
Day 10	Fruit salad Poached egg on toast	Spinach and seafood salad Wholemeal bread Fruit of choice	Chicken Juliette Jordans mixed grain Pears in burgundy

GAZPACHO
Serves 4
100g (4oz) onions
100g (4oz) cucumber, trimmed
100g (4oz) peppers, trimmed
600 ml (1pt) tomato juice
300ml (½pt) orange juice
Dash of lemon juice
60g (2½oz) fresh breadcrumbs
Dash of red wine vinegar
1 clove garlic, crushed
Salt and pepper
50g (2oz) mixed peppers, finely diced
Place roughly chopped onions, cucumber and peppers in a liquidiser and blend until smooth. Add tomato juice, orange juice, lemon juice, breadcrumbs, wine vinegar, garlic, salt and pepper. Blend well.

Chill in the fridge and serve cold, sprinkled with the diced peppers.

BEAN AND CHICKPEA SALAD
Serves 4
100g (4oz) cooked chicken breast
100g (4oz) kidney beans, soaked and cooked
100g (4oz) chickpeas, soaked and cooked
50g (2oz) leeks, finely shredded
50g (2oz) red pepper, finely shredded
50g (2oz) mushrooms, finely sliced
1 tbsp honey
1 tbsp lemon juice
Pinch of cayenne pepper
Pinch of paprika
Salt, pepper
Parsley, chopped, for garnish
Shred chicken breast. Mix together with kidney beans, chickpeas and vegetables. Add honey, lemon juice, paprika and cayenne pepper. Season and mix well, garnish with parsley.

BUTTER BEAN SOUP
Serves 4
1 meat stock cube
225g (8oz) butter beans, soaked overnight
560g (2oz) onions, chopped
25g (1oz) rosemary
1 clove garlic, crushed
900ml (1½pt) water
Salt, pepper
Pinch caraway seeds for garnish
Dissolve stock cube in water and add butter beans, onions, rosemary and garlic. Simmer until beans are tender, about 1 hour. Blend until smooth and adjust the seasoning. Garnish.

SWEDISH TROUT
Serves 4
4×150g (5oz) trout
50 g (2oz) oats
150ml (5fl oz) natural yoghurt
2 tbsp honey
2 tbsp lemon juice
2 tbsp creamed horseradish
1 eating apple, cut into small pieces
Salt and pepper
Garnish
110g (4oz) red pepper, finely diced
Parsley, chopped
Gut and clean trout. Cut off heads and fins. Roll trout in oats. Place on lightly greased baking sheet. Blend together yoghurt, honey, lemon juice and horseradish. Add apple. Season to taste, pour on four plates.

Grill trout for ten minutes and place on the beds of yoghurt sauce. Heat under the grill for one minute, being careful not to overheat as sauce will separate. Garnish.

CRISP NEW POTATOES
Serves 4
1 tbsp sunflower oil
450g (1lb) small new potatoes, scrubbed and dried
Pinch of rosemary
Salt, pepper
Preheat oven to gas mark 5 (190°C, 375°F). Heat oil in a roasting tray. Put potatoes on to a tray and coat with oil. Sprinkle with rosemary, salt and pepper. Roast for about 1 hour, until golden brown.

BAKED APPLE WITH RASPBERRIES
Serves 4
4 well-shaped cooking apples, cored
100g (4oz) brown sugar
50g (2oz) sultanas
Pinch cinnamon
4 cloves
225g (8oz) raspberries
Preheat oven to gas mark 3 (160°C, 325°F). Score around the middle of each apple. Place in an ovenproof dish. Sprinkle with sugar, sultanas, cinnamon, cloves and raspberries. Add ½ inch water. Bake for about 1 hour, basting, until golden brown.

STILTON AND HERB PATE
Serves 4
25g (1oz) butter
50g (2oz) Stilton cheese
150g (5oz) low fat cream cheese
Pinch of mixed herbs
2 tbsp chopped parsley
Salt, pepper
Garnish
4 leaves of red lettuce
12 leaves chicory
1 bunch watercress
Chopped parsley
Melt the butter in a pan, slowly stir in the Stilton, cream cheese, herbs and parsley. Season and blend together well. Chill until firm – 2 to 3 hours. Pipe pâté on the lettuce leaves and garnish.

TURKEY HELENA
Serves 4
4×110g (4oz) turkey escalopes
110g (4oz) cooked spinach
1-2 cloves garlic
50g (2oz) shelled walnuts
110g (4oz) low fat curd cheese
Salt and pepper
150ml (¼pt) chicken stock
Preheat the oven to gas mark 4 (180°C, 350°F). Remove any fat from turkey and pound the escalopes with a meat tenderiser until they are quite thin. Mince the cooked spinach and crush garlic.

Blend the spinach, garlic, walnuts and cheese together and season.

Divide the mixture into four. Place ¼ of the mixture in the middle of each escalope. Fold the turkey around the filling to form an envelope. Poach in chicken stock for 30 min in the oven. Serve with port and raspberry sauce.

FISH KEBABS WITH BROWN AND WILD RICE

Serves 4

100g (4oz) wild rice
225g (8oz) salmon
4 scallops
8 langoustines, shelled
4 red mullet, filleted
2 large red peppers trimmed
2 courgettes, trimmed
2 yellow courgettes
50ml (2fl oz) white wine
Juice of 2 lemons
1 tsp ground white pepper
25ml (1fl oz) sunflower oil
1 tsp coriander
550ml (18fl oz) fish stock
225g (8oz) brown rice
50g (2oz) parsley, chopped
Salt, pepper
Radicchio, curly endive, for garnish

Soak wild rice in cold water overnight. Cut each type of fish and seafood in eight equal rounds. Cut peppers and courgettes into rounds.

For each kebab, thread a bamboo skewer with pieces of fish and vegetable as follows: scallop, pepper, red mullet, courgette, salmon, yellow courgette, langoustine, pepper. Repeat and end with scallop.

Mix together wine, lemon juice, white pepper, oil and coriander and marinate kebabs in this mixture for up to two hours.

Pour fish stock into a saucepan and bring to the boil. Add brown and wild rice, bring back to simmering point and cover. When rice is almost cooked place the kebabs on a baking sheet and grill for 10-12 minutes, turning occasionally.

When rice is cooked, turn it out on to a baking sheet, add parsley, season to taste and mix together. Place portions of rice on to warmed plates, one kebab on each. Garnish.

TUNA COLESLAW

Serves 4

100g (4oz) white cabbage, finely shredded
25g (1oz) pineapple, chopped
1 tomato, skinned, deseeded and chopped
2 anchovy fillets, chopped finely
100g (4oz) tuna fish, canned in brine, flaked
2 tsp olive oil
2 tsp white wine vinegar
Salt, pepper
25g (1oz) chopped chives, for garnish

Mix together cabbage, pineapple, tomato, anchovies and tuna fish.

Pour oil and vinegar in a jar and season with salt and pepper. Shake until well mixed, pour over salad and toss well.

Serve with chives.

CALVES LIVER WITH RED WINE

Serves 4

350g (12oz) calves liver, in four thin slices
85ml (3fl oz) red wine
75g (3oz) tomato purée
50g (2oz) onion, chopped
25g (1oz) wholemeal flour
Salt, pepper
Broccoli florets, blanched for garnish (as in Chicken Juliette)

Preheat over to gas mark 4 (180°C, 350°F).

Dust liver with flour and fry lightly in oil until sealed. Place liver in an ovenproof dish. Sweat onions in the remaining liver juices until soft.

Pour in wine and reduce by half. Add the tomato purée and a little water, stirring well. Season and pour over the liver.

Cover and bake for 1 hour.

Arrange the liver on a plate and garnish with broccoli florets.

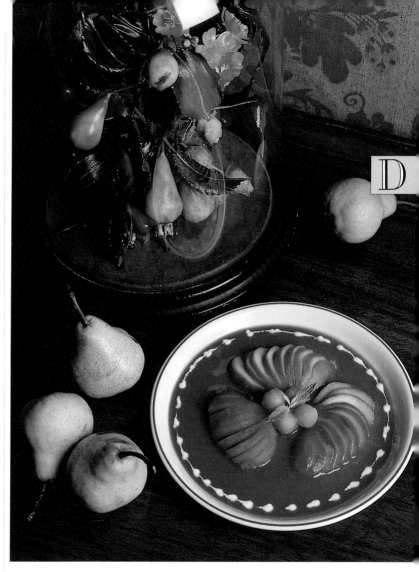

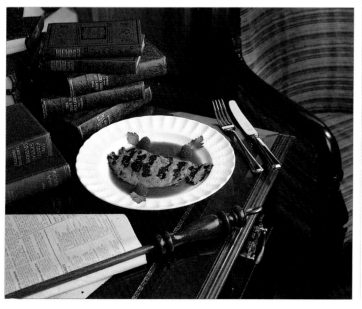

CHICKEN JULIETTE

Serves 4

600ml (1pt) chicken stock
15g (½oz) caraway seeds
4×150g (5oz) chicken breasts (skinned)
100g (4oz) carrots, peeled and chopped
100g (4oz) onions, peeled and chopped
Salt, pepper
100g (4oz) spinach, shredded
1 clove garlic, crushed
Garnish
4 small cauliflower florets
4 small broccoli florets
Parsley, chopped

Pour half the stock into frying pan. Add half of the caraway seeds and poach chicken breasts in this liquid for 30-40 minutes. Keep warm.

In another saucepan simmer carrots and half of the onion in 150ml (¼pt) of stock until soft. Then transfer to a liquidiser and blend. Season to taste.

In the last 150ml (¼pt) stock, simmer the spinach with the garlic and remaining onion for two minutes. Transfer to a liquidiser and blend. Season to taste.

Blanch cauliflower and broccoli florets by plunging into boiling water for 15 seconds and placing them in cold water immediately afterwards.

Warm plates. On to each plate pour a semicircle of each of the sauces. Place a poached chicken breast in the middle and garnish.

PEARS IN BURGUNDY

Serves 4

4 pears
225ml 8 fl oz burgundy
(50g) 2oz sugar
(25g) 1oz arrowroot
Garnish
(50g) 2oz soft exotic fruit, such as strawberries, papaya, sharon fruit

Peel the pears, leaving the stems in place. Mix wine and sugar together. Gently poach pears in the wine syrup until they are soft.

Remove the pears with a slotted spoon and leave the liquid simmering. Mix arrowroot with 2 tbsp of water, stir into the liquid and simmer for 2-3 minutes.

Slice each pear into a fan shape on a plate. Pour juice over pear fans and garnish with soft fruit.

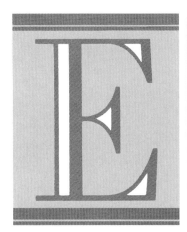

Ears

Most people have regular check-ups for teeth, eyes, heart and blood pressure – but ears miss out. We take them for granted until they start to play up. Yet the number of people suffering from hearing disorders is greater than all of those suffering from cancer, heart and kidney disease, tuberculosis, and blindness.

Fortunately many ear problems are preventable, curable and treatable. The ear is a delicate mechanism comprising the outer ear, the middle and the inner ear. Together these three chambers convert the physical pressure of sound into electrical impulses within the space of a cubic inch. Your ears feel the sound waves in the air and transmit the sensations to the brain. The inner ear also gives us a sense of balance.

Damage to any of these interrelated parts triggers hearing loss. The loss can be so gradual, people hardly notice. You may have a problem if …

You frequently turn up the television

People seem to be mumbling more than they used to

People often have to repeat what they say to you

You miss sentences or words and can't follow a conversation.

Loss of hearing can have several causes:

A severe ear infection

> Garlic and olive oil can help clear ear wax. Crush a clove of garlic in a small amount of olive oil. Heat it, not to boiling but just enough to release garlic oil into the olive oil.
>
> Sieve the liquid so that it is clear of garlic fragments. Apply two drops into the ear with a clean dropper.

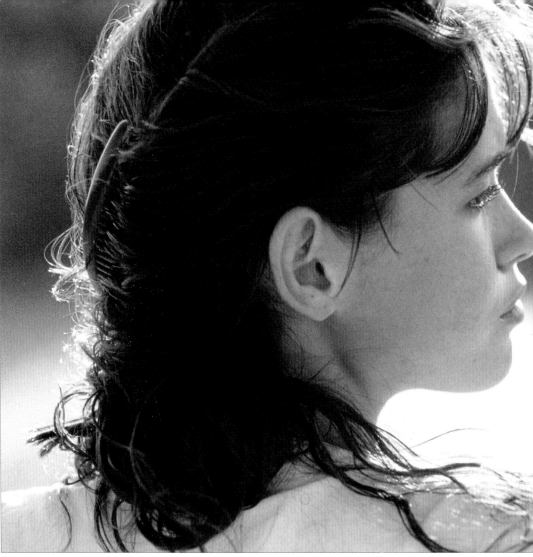

Exposure to loud noise over a prolonged period of time, such as factory noise, aeroplanes, loud music. If you have a problem hearing consonants but can hear vowels, loud noise is likely to be the cause of the problem

Age – deterioration of hearing is a consequence of ageing but need not lead to total deafness

Diet – research in Finland has shown that a low-fat diet could prevent loss of hearing, probably by keeping the blood vessels to the ears unclogged

Wax – don't try to get wax out of your ear with cotton-tipped sticks. Waxy build-up in the ear usually corrects itself through the chewing action of your jaw. There are fine little hairs in the ear which bend towards the outside, pushing wax up towards the ear's entrance. A cotton tipped swab pushes the hairs backwards preventing the normal cleansing action. If pushed too far, the swab can perforate the eardrum.

If you suspect wax is building up, see your GP. A warm water syringe will wash the wax out and is painless.

Electrolysis

This is the use of low electric current to remove hair from the legs, face and bikini line. There are two main methods:

Diathermy
A thin needle passes a current into the hair follicle's root and the cauterised hair is taken out with tweezers. Diathermy needs to be carried out several times at two-monthly intervals to get rid of all unwanted hair. There is a 20 per cent regrowth.

Galvanism
Less commonly used. A metal band is put round the wrist, or you hold a metal rod connected to the galvanic apparatus. An electric current is created when a needle is inserted in the follicle. Results are permanent.

Emotions

Emotion is expressed in the conscious mind, and also at an unconscious level of the brain where

it stimulates reflex actions in the sympathetic and parasympathetic nerves. These regulate functions such as blood flow and digestion. Emotion also affects the pituitary gland which in turn regulates other glands controlling hormonal output. (See HORMONES.)

Emotions can exacerbate and even trigger a variety of diseases. For instance, emotional upset can precipitate an asthma attack, causing a reflex spasm of the muscle fibres in the walls of the air passages in the lungs. Skin disorders such as eczema and digestive disorders including over-eating, duodenal ulcers, irritable bowel syndrome, as well as migraine and high blood pressure can all be attributed to emotion that is inappropriately handled.

The British are particularly inept at dealing with emotions; the stiff upper lip mentality prefers to repress rather than express. From an early age most of us learn to suppress our tears or anger, or to rationalise our strongest feelings and needs because it is considered unseemly to act as emotions dictate. This repression of

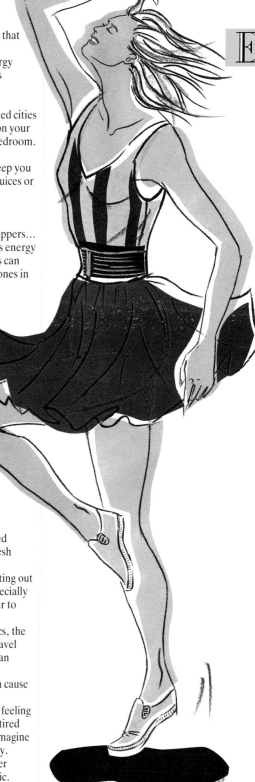

E

physical responses to emotion, such as crying or shouting, can in time lead to physical and psychological illness.

A person can learn not to punch someone on the nose whenever he is angry, but he cannot stop his pulse racing, the increased working of his adrenal glands, and the many other physical adjustments going on inside his body. Repressing his anger will in time lead to physical illness, and can cause DEPRESSION.

This is not to say that anyone feeling angry should immediately punch someone on the nose! There are ways of expressing anger which are not physically harmful to anyone. Acknowledging and expressing how we feel heals ourselves and our relationships, but we may hold back out of fear of rejection and hurt, or of being overwhelmed by our emotions and losing control. Overcoming these fears is the first step to emotional health.

⬤ Always say what's on your mind at the time, rather than bottling it up.

⬤ Share feelings of sadness and fear with others, rather than deny them or keeping them secret.

⬤ Identify the cause of sadness, grief, hurt. Express your feelings in relation to the cause.

⬤ Find outlets for anger and aggression that are not harmful. Try physical exercise, kicking a ball, punching a pillow, shouting as loud as you can.

⬤ Meditation may help you recognise and accept parts of yourself you are trying to hide. COUNSELLING may help you get in touch with your emotions.

ENERGY

The sun is the ultimate source of all energy. It powers every part of our lives, from the oxygen we breathe in to the plants and animals that feed us. This energy is converted by our bodies via a series of complex chemical changes into the energy that fuels our actions and emotions. (See CALORIES.)

Just as a well serviced and maintained engine will use fuel economically, a healthy body is crucial for the efficient production and use of its energy.

And the more energy you have, the more enthusiasm you can put into your everyday routine. Energy brings big rewards.

GET UP AND GO

Want to start the day bouncing out of bed, instead of lying there wishing you never had to get up? Close your eyes, take long, slow deep breaths. You'll be taking in extra doses of oxygen, the body's energiser. (See BREATHING/RELAXATION.) Feel yourself relaxing, imagine the sun, its golden rays warming every part of your body. See yourself doing your everyday chores filled with this energising radiance.

Return to the image of the sun, this time shining over a favourite landscape. Open eyes, get up slowly. Notice how light and energised you feel.

Then try a 'sunny' breakfast. Fresh juice from fruits that have ripened in the sun; a poached or boiled egg, its yolk like a full rising sun, two slices of wholewheat toast with grains that you can see.

ENERGY BOOSTERS

Take a walk. A ten-minute brisk walk beats after-lunch lethargy. Studies have shown that walkers report lower tension levels and higher energy levels for as long as two hours after their stroll.

Ionisers can help you feel energised, especially in polluted cities and offices. Keep an ioniser on your desk, in the car and in your bedroom. (See IONS.)

Resist drinking coffee to keep you going. Drink mineral water, juices or herbal teas instead.

ENEMIES OF ENERGY

Watch out for these energy sappers...

⬤ A sedentary lifestyle lowers energy levels. Take up aerobics – this can boost mood-improving hormones in the brain that make you feel revitalised and improves the quality of sleep and appetite.

⬤ Energy drops just before and during menstruation. Listen to your body and be easy on yourself – don't overwork. And eat lots of iron-rich food such as spinach and liver. Be kind to yourself and energy levels will soon rise.

⬤ Bad eating habits – a DIET overloaded with fat and refined carbohydrates, not enough fresh vegetables and fruit.

⬤ Beat sleepless nights by cutting out caffeine. Restrict alcohol, especially before bedtime. Allow an hour to unwind before bed.

⬤ Anti-depressants, antibiotics, the contraceptive pill and some travel sickness pills and painkillers can cause tiredness.

⬤ Avoid crash diets – they can cause low energy levels.

⬤ You can think yourself into feeling tired. We often expect to feel tired after a day's work, but try to imagine yourself feeling fresh and lively. POSITIVE THINKING is a healthier pick-me-up than a gin and tonic.

⬤ Tiredness may be related to certain foods or chemicals. (See ALLERGIES.)

⬤ Smoking tires the body by depleting the body's supply of energy-producing oxygen. There's only one way to regain the levels of energy lost from years of smoking – give up!

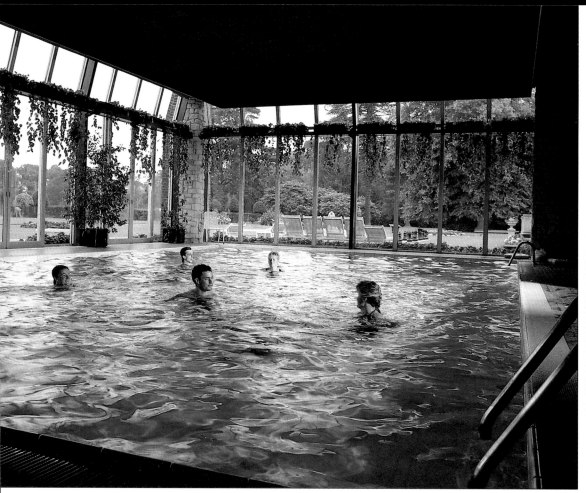

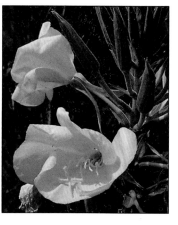

● Hangovers
● Premenstrual Syndrome
(See PMS)
● Prevention of heart attacks – the oil is believed to contain an anti-clotting factor
● Skin conditions such as eczema

The oil is available in capsules or in liquid form from pharmacists and health stores. The only other sources of GLA are human breast milk and fish.

EXERCISE

If the idea of spending 30 minutes a day exercising seems a boring chore and you would only consider it if you have put on a few extra pounds, then think again…

The human body is designed to move – not just shift in a chair several times a day – but *really* move! The more you put your body through its paces, the stronger, healthier and more co-ordinated it gets.

You benefit mentally and psychologically too; regular strenuous exercise frees the body from its habitual daily restrictions and allows it to express itself. A daily swim is ideal.

Some exercise converts describe a newfound sense of well-being – suddenly almost anything seems possible! There are many reasons why people incorporate exercise into their lives. Some want to lose weight, or improve their body shape, others want to increase their energy levels or simply stay healthy and fit. However, exercise alone does not guarantee health. A body that is battling with an ill-balanced diet, cigarettes and alcohol cannot reap the full benefits of regular exercise. (Although studies show that exercising does help people give up smoking and encourages a healthier appetite.)

You don't have to join a health club to keep fit or spend a lot of money on

ESSENTIAL OILS

Essential oils are the basic materials of AROMATHERAPY. The highly aromatic essences of flowers, bark, roots, stems and resins are extracted mainly by distillation. Highly concentrated, they are rarely used undiluted. A few drops are added to a carrier oil, such as almond or olive oil, and massaged into the skin to be absorbed through the pores. They can be added to BATHING water or inhaled through steam, but

---

Same aromatherapists make up these toners to keep skin sparkling!

For oily skin
4 drops blue camomile
10 ml vodka
250 ml distilled water

For normal skin
250 ml rose-water
15 ml vodka
3 drops Palmarosa
3 drops rose

For dry skin
250 ml rose-water
10 ml vodka
4 drops rose absolute
2 drops Roman camomile

---

should never be taken internally.

Essential oils are used for both beauty and health. They are believed to have the power to sedate or uplift, and provide relief in a wide range of chronic conditions, such as rheumatoid arthritis, mental illness, gallstones and bronchitis. Some oils like fennel and geranium contain plant hormones similar to the female hormone oestrogen and can help keep the face looking young, as well as promoting a balance for the menstrual cycle.

All oils are chemically complex and highly volatile. They are mainly colourless or pale yellow and are easily damaged by ultraviolet light. They should be stored in opaque bottles away from direct sunlight. The oils also react to extremes of temperature and vibrations.

Essential oils can be purchased from an aromatherapist and some pharmacies and health stores, but before using them consult a qualified aromatherapist. Small amounts of some essential oils can build up to a toxic level in the body, and some of the oils are poisonous, so follow the aromatherapist's instructions carefully.

For instance, for respiratory problems – add three drops of lavender oil to a bowl of steaming

water. Put a towel over your head and around the bowl and inhale for ten minutes. Do this first thing in the morning, around midday and before bedtime.

For MASSAGE, add three or four drops of your recommended essential oil to a carrier oil – almond, sunflower or sesame – and massage gently into the skin.

EVENING PRIMROSE OIL

Evening Primrose grows wild and its long spikes of luminous yellow petals open only at night. The oil is expressed from the flower's tiny seeds and contains a high level of gamma linolenic acid (GLA) – an essential fatty acid used by the body to manufacture hormone-like substances called prostaglandins. The healthy functioning of many types of body tissue is helped by these prostaglandins, which limit inflammatory reactions.

Current research suggests that Evening Primrose Oil is beneficial for the following:
● Arthritis
● Brittle finger nails
● Coughing
● Cramp

clothes and equipment. Exercise can be done at home in the garden, at work or even while you are commuting.

Any exercise programme should include relaxation and stretching movements and take individual needs into account. For example, if you tend to put on weight, consider a prolonged steady type of exercise such as golf, walking, swimming. Newcomers to exercise, or older people, should avoid anything that involves sudden, jarring movements, such as jogging. Ask yourself whether you prefer a social activity (golf, tennis) or solitude (swimming), and why you want to exercise – to build up stamina (running, swimming) or strength (weightlifting) or both? If you suffer from high blood pressure, are recuperating from an illness, suffer dizzy spells and get out of breath easily, check with your doctor first. Always start exercising gently. Don't try to prove you're superman or superwoman. You could seriously injure yourself.

You don't need to set aside a specific time to exercise. It can be incorporated into your working day...
A daily walk to or from the station can add to your weekly mileage.
A lunchtime walk of ¾ mile will also be beneficial. If that's impossible, take an evening walk.
Use the stairs instead of the lift. If you are so out of condition that one flight leaves you exhausted, try a few steps at a time before resting, adding three steps each day, until you can manage to climb three

E

	ADVANTAGES	DISADVANTAGES	TIPS
AEROBICS	Can be done at home or in a class Sociable, fun Good cardiovascular exercise	If incorrectly taught can lead to injuries Need to rely on a class Lonely at home	Buy special shoes Floor must not be solid concrete Make sure instructor is qualified
CYCLING	Easily incorporated into daily life. Apart from bike, no other expense Excellent strength and aerobic exercise if cycling consistently	If in town, exposes lungs to car fumes Traffic dangers	When winter cycling becomes unpleasant, switch to exercise bike Learn Highway Code Wear a reflective chest band
DANCE	Fun Good for strength and flexibility Creative	Risk of muscular injuries Not always aerobic, depends on the type of dancing	Join a class where you have same abilities
FIXED WEIGHT TRAINING (Multigym, Nautilus etc)	Safer than free weights Good for firming and toning Highly specific – can concentrate on weak muscles	Expensive to do at home Need special facilities Lonely, boring	Try out equipment first Build up gradually For aerobic benefit keep weight light, allow multiple repetitions
FREE WEIGHT TRAINING (dumbbells etc)	Firms and tones muscles Can use at home	Risk of injury if not supervised	Over 35s – check for high blood pressure Learn proper lifting techniques Use as adjunct to an aerobic activity
FOOTBALL	Good exercise Sociable Cheap	Risk of injury Depends on finding fellow players	Five-a-side football gives maximum fitness
RUNNING & JOGGING	Good aerobic exercise Shoes are the only expense Don't need special facilities See progress at a weekly rate	Can overdo it Risk of injuries to feet, ankles, knees and hips. Overweight are especially vulnerable. Can be boring	Women shouldn't run alone Build up training gradually Change route to beat boredom Run on soft surfaces Buy good running shoes
SKIING	Good for strength and flexibility Sociable	High risk of injury Unless skilled, little aerobic benefit Expensive	Develop a pre-ski programme Use dry ski run regularly
SWIMMING	Uses every major muscle in the body Low injury risk Not weight-bearing, so good if pregnant, overweight, elderly or disabled Good for flexibility and strength	Swimming facilities may not be easily accessible Boring Chlorine can damage hair and dry skin	A weight-bearing exercise is also advisable Mix strokes for maximum benefit Use an all-over moisturiser after swimming
TENNIS	Low injury risk Sociable Excitement of competition Good for general fitness	Unless played at high level little aerobic value Can be expensive Depends on finding fellow player	Join a club with indoor facilities Singles maximises exercise
WALKING	Cheap and easy daily routine Low injury risk Excellent aerobic activity if brisk	Easy to slow down when not thinking	For maximum benefit pace has to be consistently brisk Breathe deeply while walking

flights all in one go.

While waiting for a train or taxi, strengthen calf muscles by raising heels from the ground and take your weight on your toes. Hold for the count of seven and lower heels. Repeat ten times.

Next, pull your abdomen in towards the spine, clench fists, tense thigh muscles, count to ten and then relax.

Repeat with all the major muscles ten times.

EXFOLIATORS

Exfoliators, scrubs and sloughing lotions basically consist of granules suspended in a gel or lotion to scrub off dead cells and grime, and leave skin smoother and clearer. Used regularly, they keep blemishes and blackheads at bay and stimulate circulation. Rubbed gently all over the body, an exfoliant can tone the skin. Rinse off the granules with a warm shower followed by splashes of cold water.

If your skin is sensitive or very fair, it's wise to give exfoliators a miss. Gentle rubbing with a damp flannel followed by a massage with a moisturiser can be just as effective. For men, exfoliants used before a shave will help to prevent ingrown facial hairs.

Sea salt is an effective body exfoliator. Sprinkle over damp flannel and massage over the skin after a warm bath, shower off and follow with a brisk towel rub. The drying effect of salt should be counteracted by a rich moisturising cream or lotion. Do not rub salt on the face.

Do not massage vigorously with exfoliators – the tiny granules can scratch and break the skin. Most exfoliators should not be used more than once a week.

EYES

The eyes are not only the windows of the soul, but also reveal the body's state of health.

A doctor can tell whether a patient is suffering from diabetes or brain tumours just by looking into the eyes with a beam of light. An iridologist claims to be able to diagnose all sorts of mineral and vitamin deficiencies and diseases by examining the irises. (See IRIDOLOGY.)

It isn't actually your eyes that see, it's your brain. The messages received by the eye in the form of

light patterns are passed on to a layer of photosensitive cells at the back of the eyeball called the retina. The patterns travel by a nerve impulse via the optic nerve to the brain where they are immediately transformed into the image we see.

Current research shows that light is a major contributor to maintaining good general health. Via the retina, light stimulates the body's major glands, the pineal and pituitary glands affecting our body chemistry and hormonal balance. The exposure of the naked eye to ultraviolet wavelengths in the open air has been discovered to affect our energy levels and emotions, but nowadays we spend more and more time indoors under artificial lighting. So make a point of spending at least an hour a day out of doors.

Some eye problems are caused by vitamin and mineral deficiencies...

A diet with adequate vitamin A is essential for eye health. Night blindness is the first sign of vitamin A deficiency. Extra doses were given to pilots on night raids in World War II. Fresh apricots, carrots, broccoli, liver, spinach, sweet potatoes, kale and lettuce all contain vitamin A.

Watering eyes and lids that feel gritty on the eye could indicate a deficiency of vitamin B2 (found in almonds, brewer's yeast, cheese, chicken, wheatgerm, liver, kidney). But the most likely causes are lack of sleep and a smoky atmosphere.

A lack of B9 (in lentils, oranges, liver, green leafy vegetables) dims vision. A healthy intake of the B complex vitamins helps to ensure healthy eye function and keeps fine skin around eyes smooth and supple.

Vitamin C is believed to protect the eye lens against chemicals normally produced by the action of light. A high concentration of vitamin C is found in the lens and the fluid between the lens and

the cornea.

One of the highest concentrations of zinc in the body occurs in the retina of the eye and zinc is also essential for the body's absorption of vitamin A. (Zinc is found in egg yolk, derived milk, pork, wheat bran, wholegrain products, lean beef, sesame seeds.)

EYES RIGHT

Don't short-change your eyes. Make sure lighting in your workplace and home is adequate. Avoid glare from unprotected light bulbs, or bright light reflecting on a window or shiny surfaces.

Don't spend long hours staring at a VDU screen. Staring at the screen slows down your blinking rate and dries eyes. Give yourself a ten-minute break every hour.

If eyes feel strained, splash them with warm water, preferably containing sea salt.

To ease puffiness around the eyes, gently massage with eye gel containing natural ingredients such as elderflower, marigold, camomile and witch-hazel.

Puffiness may also be caused by premenstrual water retention. On waking apply cool compresses such as ice cubes wrapped in cloth, or cucumber or potato slices.

Any puffiness accompanied by redness, pain and tenderness should be reported to your doctor.

If you suffer from cold sores, be very careful not to touch your face and then your eyes. The herpes virus can be very damaging to your sight. If you see a doctor because your eye is inflamed, always mention if you have had a cold sore. Otherwise steroid drops or ointment may be prescribed, which in the case of inflammation caused by herpes can permanently scar your eyes unless you are given an antiviral injection.

Have an eye test once a year. (See GLASSES, CONTACT LENSES.)

For extra eye power try these exercises...

Blink quickly – about 50 times per minute.

In the morning splash closed eyes 20 times with warm water, then 20 times with cold. Repeat at bedtime, reversing the sequence.

For a few minutes at intervals during the day, cover your eyes with the palms of the hands, placing the bases of the little fingers on the bridge of the nose. This rests your eyes.

With your head held still and eyes open, look upwards, then to the right, downwards, and to the left. Feel the eye muscles working. Repeat five times, then roll the eyes round full circle.

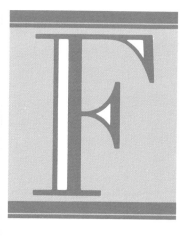

FACE

That old expression 'It's written all over your face' highlights one of the functions of all those muscles that lie beneath the surface of the face. They tug and pull at the skin to create a wide range of signals which communicate how you feel – for instance, it's the muscles that actively move the skin around the eyes to create an expression, not the eyes themselves. Your mouth, too, is tugged up and down either to smile or grimace. When lips tighten, muscles are usually responding to anxiety or anger.

Tune into your facial expressions and understand yourself better. A knowledge of your partner's repertoire of emotionally charged facial expressions can often help avert a crisis. Facial signals relating to a particular emotion are frequently given out before the feeling is verbalised.

A psychologist at the University of Connecticut in USA has found that people who consistently express themselves visually are under less physiological tension than other people and may put their bodies under less stress during their lifetime.

FACING UP TO IT

The skin on your face is – apart from your hands – the most exposed area on your body, so it needs to be well looked after.

Use a humidifier or place a dish of water on top of a radiator in your workplace and at home to add moisture to the atmosphere. Central heating dehydrates the skin.

Always wear a sunscreen – whether on holiday or not – to protect skin from the sun's damaging rays.

Smoking puckers skin around the lips permanently – especially on women.

Men and women should use a moisturising cream daily and avoid

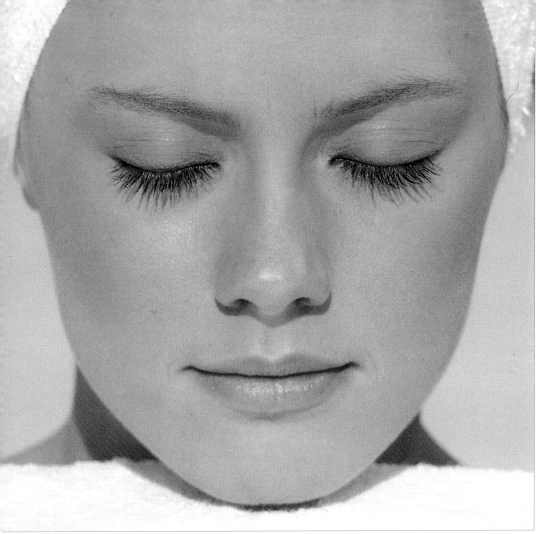

electrical treatments . . .

● Hi-frequency treatments are excellent for refining and cleansing oily skins. The gentle germicidal action works on spots and mild acne.

● Galvanic treatments, such as cathiodermie, are more stimulating. Gels are selected to suit your skin type, massaged into the skin and then absorbed with the help of the electric current relayed through rollers passing over the skin. (Electricity has been used in beauty for 50 years – the normal electrical current is modified and very safe.)

Most facials tend to follow a basic step-by-step routine:

● Cleanse – to unclog pores and wipe away accumulated grime (can be steam or lotions)

● Tone – to invigorate skin

● Peel or scrub – remove dead cells

● Massage – to improve blood circulation and stimulate removal of lymphatic waste

● Mask – to nourish and soften skin, moisturise, protect, soothe and soften. (See MASK)

The ingredients of a facial will be chosen to suit your skin type. For instance, if you have a dry, mature skin there are plenty of beauty lotions, ampoules and gels containing extracts of herbs, seaweed or algae that will plump out tissues to smooth out surface wrinkles. The youthful effect lasts for about a week.

You may have a facial using only hypo-allergenic products which are

F

using harsh astringents. The skin around the eyes is particularly delicate.

FACE LIFT
Facial muscles tend to be overlooked, but they work hard and gather a lot of tension during the day. Regular massage can relieve tensions.

Here's how . . .

● Smooth a little oil or massage cream over skin so fingertips can glide easily.

● Clear puffiness around the eyes by massaging the valley above the collar bone.

● Place fingers in centre of forehead from brow up to hairline. Press firmly to count of three, then release. Move fingers apart by half an inch, and repeat.

Finish with fingertips on hairline at the temple.

● Place fingertips under the eyes pressing gently, turn inwards to press down along the bridge of the nose to the corners of the mouth. Repeat the movement several times around mouth.

● Place fingers like a fan under cheekbones. Press and release,

continuing the movement down to the jawline.

● Place palms of hands flat against neck with fingers behind the ears and circle five times.

● Apply hot and cold COMPRESSES to remove impurities. Gently remove oil or massage cream, then repeat with cold compress.

FACIALS

Treat yourself at least once a month to a facial and see what a difference it makes to your skin and sense of well-being.

There are so many different facials now available it can be confusing. A beauty therapist will be able to recommend a treatment that is best suited to your skin type, but generally facials fall into four categories – deep cleansing, rejuvenating, nourishing or hypo-allergenic.

If you live and work in an urban area, it's likely your skin will need a regular spring clean! To lift the dirt out of the pores effectively there is now a wide range of deep-cleansing

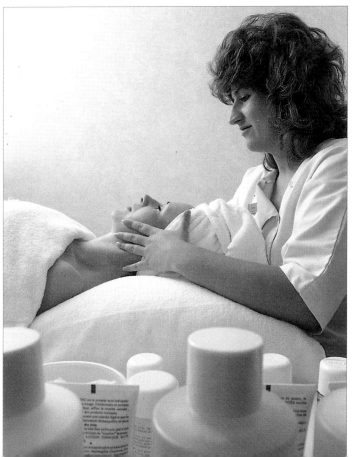

deep-cleansing and nourishing, but which include no perfumes or known irritants.

A facial massage is not always included, but is worth having. It gets to the neck and shoulders, which are often two of the body's worst tension spots.

FARADIC EXERCISE

Faradic exercise equipment, such as Slendertone, works on the principle that you don't have to move a muscle – the machine does it all for you. Electrode attachments are placed on specific points of the body and face and a mild electric current automatically contracts the muscles. It is safe and is recommended for post plastic surgery patients to restore muscle strength and tone up facial muscles.

Faradic exercise is ideal for spot reducing, as it can be focused on one particular area and is particularly effective in tightening fat tummies.

This form of exercise should only be considered along with other types of exercise, eg AEROBIC. It is not recommended if you have just had a baby.

Treatments usually last 20 minutes and can be taken once or twice a week. After a course of eight treatments you should see results.

FASTING

Controlled fasting has been used as a form of therapy for more than 2,000 years. Hippocrates, the father of modern medicine, used it as a treatment for some diseases in the belief that it allowed the body to concentrate all its resources on dealing with the disease. Most sick animals instinctively refuse food until the body's healing mechanisms have

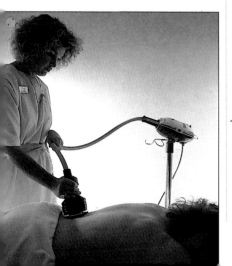

done their work.

Fasting at home should not last longer than 48 hours. Supervised fasts, for instance at a health resort, can be undertaken for longer periods.

Fasts encourage weight loss, but were originally intended as a means of general detoxification. There is a sense of well-being after a fast – the body feels purified and energised – but there can also be unpleasant side effects such as nausea, hair loss, dry skin, muscle cramps, fatigue, depression, bad breath and irritability.

Certain people should not fast including pregnant and pre-menstrual women, and people recuperating from an illness.

48-HOUR FAST RULES
● Begin the fast the night before by having a light meal such as a salad, a bowl of natural live yoghurt, fruit or a clear soup.
● Drink between four and eight pints of mineral or distilled water during the fast. Add a teaspoon of vitamin C (ascorbic acid) to each quart of water.
● Liquid should be consumed at roughly two hour intervals. Take plenty of rest – avoid exertion.
● Don't drive – you often feel light-headed during a fast.
● Slight nausea and headaches may occur. If you are taking any medications, do not fast without consulting your doctor.
● Avoid smoking.
● The first meal after a fast should be a light one, such as vegetable soup or yoghurt.

FATIGUE

After pain, fatigue is the second most common complaint in the doctor's surgery.

Fatigue severely reduces people's ability to function. It is normal to be tired after a great deal of mental or physical exertion, but if tiredness is apparent at inappropriate times, such as after a rest, a sufferer's quality of life is being drastically affected.

You need to explore a number of areas in your life to uncover reasons for extreme tiredness. Have a close look at your current lifestyle, emotional relationships, diet, work, environmental pollution, drug usage, past health history, exercise, habits and attitudes, menstrual cycle. Very often it can take just a small change in your lifestyle to restore energy, such as learning a relaxation technique to help combat stress, taking up exercise, cutting out coffee, giving up

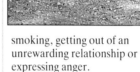

smoking, getting out of an unrewarding relationship or expressing anger.

Note when the fatigue began and what your circumstances were at the time. Had there been any major changes in your life? Did you include a new food in your diet? You could be allergic to it. Do you recall any illness which preceded the onset of your fatigue by six to 12 months?

Keep a fatigue diary – write down details about each onset of fatigue, the weather, meals, activity, company, how long it lasts. Note other symptoms associated with fatigue such as headache, hunger, indigestion. Does your fatigue prevent you from doing what you don't want to do anyway?

The diary should be able to give you some indication of your personal fatigue factors. You may need to supplement your diet with certain vitamins, minerals or amino acids. You may need to exercise more often. Regular massage might help to ease away body tension – another cause of extreme tiredness.

Fatigue is not a natural state. Tuning into your body and lifestyle is the first step to fighting it.

FATS

Contrary to popular opinion, fat is actually good for you! It keeps you warm, stores energy, keeps skin and arteries supple, protects from heart disease and allergies, and balances hormones. It's *how much* fat you eat that makes the difference. Eat

too much and you risk strokes, heart attacks, breast cancer, diabetes, gallstones. It is recommended that the body should get no more than 30 per cent of its calories from fat, but the average Western intake is 42 per cent. Just as important is the type of fat you eat.

Saturated fat – usually solid at room temperature and occurring mainly in animal foods. If you are eating enough CARBOHYDRATE foods, like grains, beans, lentils and fruits, you can cut down on saturated fats. Avocado, coconut, eggs, cheese, pork and beef all contain a high level of saturated fats.

Polyunsaturated fats – usually in the form of vegetable oils such as sunflower and in nuts, seeds and fish. We have been encouraged to include plenty of polyunsaturates in our diet because they are shown to reduce cholesterol levels in the blood, minimising coronary heart disease – but they should still be used with moderation. An overall reduction in saturated fats should not be accompanied by an increase in polyunsaturated fats.

Mono-unsaturated fat – recent medical research shows that mono-unsaturated fat aids efficient working of the heart. Main sources are olive oil and fish.

Essential fatty acids (EFA) – known as Vitamin F, EFA are essential for health. The two important EFAs are linoleic acid and linolenic acid found in polyunsaturated fats in game, meat, grains, vegetables and EVENING PRIMROSE OIL.

Cholesterol – much maligned, but is essential for hormone and bile

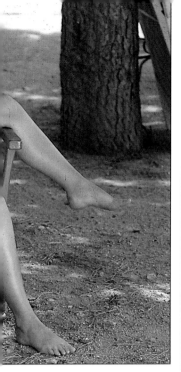

production and is contained in every cell in the body. It's a waxy, insoluble substance that is manufactured in the body and is found in animal fats and eggs. Levels in the blood build up when the diet is high in refined CARBOHYDRATES, saturated fats and sugar, leading to heart disease.

FEET

Feet are often the most neglected part of the body. We cram them into tight-fitting shoes and march up and down on them all day. It's time our feet were liberated!

Try and walk barefoot around the house whenever you can, and give yourself a home pedicure at least once a week:

● Soak feet for 15 minutes in warm water with a few drops of almond oil.
● Dry thoroughly and push cuticles back if necessary with a stick wrapped in cotton wool.
● Clip nails straight across.
● Smooth any calluses with a foot file or pumice stone. Don't cut hard skin yourself.
● Massage feet gently with body or foot cream, cover with warm towels for ten minutes and relax.

If you spend a lot of time on your feet during the day, try a footbath in the evening – add three drops of an essential oil to a bowl of hot water. Marjoram, lavender and rosemary all help relieve overworked muscles.

The choice of footwear for children will determine whether or not their feet will be healthy in adult life…

● Avoid fitted footwear for children

until they are about two years old. Until then let them run around in thick socks or barefoot.
● Choose a shoe that is supple and light and does not distort their toes. There must be room for big toes to point forwards.
● Review their footwear regularly.
● Teenagers should avoid high heels (above 3 cm) until they are at least 18. High shoes pitch the body forward, ramming feet into the front of the shoes and deforming them.

FIBRE

Fibre, the outer fibrous coat of grain, plays a crucial role in the digestive system. Wheat, barley, oats, rye, maize and rice all consist of a starchy middle with a fibrous bran coat in their unrefined state.

Fibre helps food travel faster through the intestine and makes stools softer, preventing constipation and damage to the intestine walls, and clears out lurking waste. Studies show that it slows down the absorption of sugars – preventing high blood sugar levels, protects against gallstones, reduces cholesterol levels, rectal and colon cancer.

Fibre is found mostly in unrefined carbohydrates such as plant foods, whole grains, vegetables and fruit. A balanced diet should contain a minimum of 30 per cent fibre. To top up your daily intake, sprinkle bran on breakfast cereals, or add a spoonful to soups and stews.

FITNESS

Be fit for anything! Feel healthy, strong, supple and in control of your life. A fit body is one that exercises regularly, and is fuelled by a balanced diet containing plenty of fibre, fresh vegetables and fruit. (See DIET.)

Being fit means that you're more likely to wake up in the morning looking forward to what the new day will bring. You can work hard during the day but still have plenty of energy for fun in the evening. You will look terrific and people will respond to you in a positive way. A fit person knows that whatever problems the day throws up they will be able to meet them head on.

To get fit you have to be willing to break away from the crowd. Lots of people eat chocolate and snack on junk food when time is pressing, so why shouldn't you? Because

getting fit is a positive step – it takes time and effort – and you need to discover the benefits for yourself.

The first step towards fitness is understanding how your body works and how you can maximise its potential.

Find out as much as you can about your body and its responses. Draw up a healthy balanced diet and see what changes you have to make to accommodate it.

Trying new dishes and discovering new tastes is exciting.

If you smoke, find out what effect all that nicotine and carbon monoxide has on you and those around you. It's a major barrier to all-round fitness.

The bonus of being fit is that you will be less susceptible to unhealthy cravings – for cigarettes, sugar or coffee. They will be replaced by a healthy appetite that wants only the best for the body it is fuelling.

FLUID RETENTION

Fluid retention in the body usually causes swelling of the feet, ankles and abdomen, and indicates a sluggish LYMPHATIC SYSTEM. It is more likely to occur in women, especially before menstruation.

A long plane journey can produce swelling of the ankles and more generalised fluid retention may result in swollen fingers and puffiness around the eyes.

Fluid retention is uncomfortable and makes most sufferers feel bloated and lacking in confidence, but there are measures you can take to help reduce it:

● Steer clear of salt – it helps retain body fluid.
● Ignore refined CARBOHYDRATES. They require a lot of water to be metabolised. By cutting them out you will find yourself rushing off to the toilet more often – a sure sign that the body isn't retaining water any longer!
● Avoid diuretics (water tablets). In the short term they reduce fluid retention, but in the long term fluid is increased as the body adjusts to the biochemical changes they cause. Fluid retention will get worse when the diuretic is stopped, but will soon settle down. Settle for natural diuretics instead, such as celery and water melon.
● Check for food allergies. Women who suffer pre-menstrual fluid retention often have an intolerance to wheat, grain, yeast or dairy products.

● If diet is unbalanced take vitamin B6 (up to 100mg per day but not for more than three months) and a supplement of magnesium, or increase your intake of wholegrain cereals, bananas and wheatgerm.
● Add six drops of caraway essential oil to a warm bath. Caraway is a stimulant and diuretic.

Or try three drops of rosemary oil in your bath and relax for ten blissful minutes.
● This may seem paradoxical, but drink plenty of mineral water – it flushes out unwanted fluids!

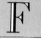

FLYING

The biggest problem for air travellers is dehydration. Pressurised cabin air is very dry so apply a good moisturiser to the skin before and during the flight. This applies to both men and women.

Contact lens wearers should either take their lenses out before the flight, or use special drops to keep their eyes moist.

Avoid alcohol before and during the flight as it increases dehydration. Cabin pressure also reduces the liver's ability to process alcohol. In flight hangovers are three times worse than on the ground. Drink plenty of mineral water instead.

Don't smoke! Book a seat well away from the smokers' area. Cabin pressure increases the absorption of carbon monoxide in cigarette smoke, so can cause headaches and lethargy.

Sitting for long periods affects circulation and encourages fluid retention. Avoid drinking tea and coffee in a plane, because they are stimulants and will not help you to relax.

Wear loose fitting clothing and a pair of slippers – feet swell, particularly on a long flight. Try and rest with your feet up if possible. Move around as often as you can.

Use a soothing eye gel to reduce any puffiness around the eyes. (See JET LAG.)

Make up a flight bag and keep on permanent standby. It should contain: eye pads, eye gel, contact lens solution (if required), moisturiser, slippers, mouth freshener/mints, inflatable pillow, ear plugs, tissues, two handkerchiefs each sprinkled separately with rosemary and sandalwood. Sniff sandalwood before take-off – it helps you relax. Rosemary will help combat mental fatigue, so sniff that one before landing.

FUN!

Adults need to have as much fun as children. Play relaxes, stimulates and brings laughter into our lives – all very valuable ingredients for positive health. (See LAUGHTER.)

Fun in life often seems to dwindle as soon as we take on the responsibilities of adulthood. To bring back its thrill and delight we need to get in touch with the child in us – so often forgotten in the rush to 'grow up'.

One simple reason why adults enjoy spending time with children is because it allows them to have some fun and games; a child's natural joy and enthusiasm for life is infectious – it can rub off and make a stressed adult suddenly feel a lot healthier.

Having fun isn't being childish, it's being child*like*, and there's an enormous difference between the two. Maturity is knowing when and where certain kinds of behaviour are appropriate, and being able to recognise a good playmate – someone who will allow your playful side to show without being patronising or judgmental.

Having fun is a wonderful way of releasing stress. It means we bring laughter into our lives, and for a while drop all the masks of adulthood – of self-importance and concern for appearances – that inhibit us. So indulge the child in you. Renew your capacity for wonder, the love of learning, the ability to play.

Youngsters will put you in touch with the child in you – so will animals. Dolphins at play, for example, are a joy to watch. If you think that sounds crazy, try it.

Spend time with those friends who enjoy sharing their sense of fun with you. Notice how much more emotionally open they are than those who think fun is child's play or demeaning. Fun people smile more often, too. Sport is a good source of fun, if not taken too seriously.

Remember that holidays shouldn't be the only time when you set out to have fun; you can spontaneously and easily incorporate fun into your daily life if you allow that child within you out to play. Kick off your shoes and run barefoot through the park. Have a snowball fight. Wrestle with your lover and see who wins. Have a pillow fight with the kids. Build a sandcastle. Be a fun person!

Release that unabashed love of fun with its lack of concern for appearances and self-importance.

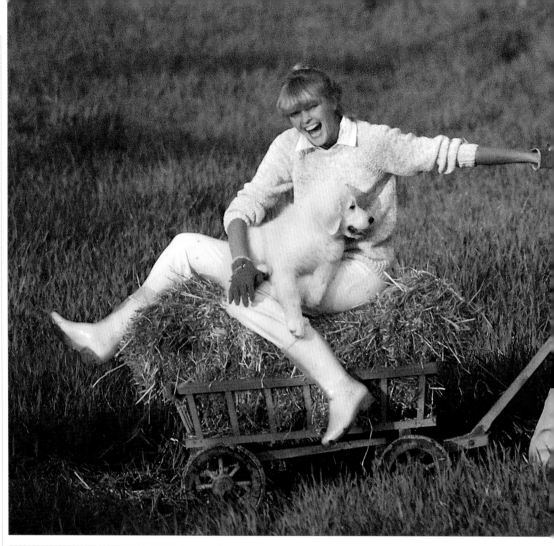

GARLIC

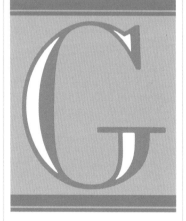

Ancient folklore insists that garlic will keep vampires at bay. Not surprising, considering its strong, lingering smell! It is also one of the most widely used plants in the world, both in the kitchen and for healing.

As one of nature's most powerful antiseptic oils, garlic is being increasingly recognised as effective in preventing high blood pressure and heart disease. It also reduces cholesterol levels and can help in the treatment of bronchitis, sinusitis and catarrh as well as gastro-intestinal infections. It's also well known for its libido-boosting qualities – pity about the smelly breath!

Garlic has a high sulphur content which can help skin infections and acne.

If the smell of garlic is too strong for you and your friends, take it in capsule form, or chew a pinch of parsley or coffee beans after eating. Henry IV was baptised with a clove of garlic rubbed on the tongue, followed by a spoonful of armagnac to prepare him for any of life's challenges!

If you include garlic in your life each day, you'll be protecting your body against a wide range of infections and diseases.

GINSENG

The restorative qualities of ginseng are legendary and it has been used in the East, especially China and Korea, for thousands of years. Ginseng may counteract fatigue and depression and has gained a reputation as an aphrodisiac.

As ginseng is such a powerful stimulant, it is important not to overuse it. Up to 1,200mg a day can be taken in capsule form for up to three weeks after periods of physical or mental crisis, otherwise keep intake to 600mg a day during convalescence or to combat tiredness.

GLASSES

Visual deterioration is often so gradual it is hardly noticed. An annual eye test will reveal any problems. If you don't need glasses in your early 20s, your eyesight is likely to remain stable until your early 40s. (See EYES.)

There is now such an enormous range of styles in glasses that it's often difficult to choose. Here's how *not* to make a spectacle of yourself:
● Smile! If frames move it's because they're resting on your cheeks. Choose a shallower pair.
● Glasses should be no wider than

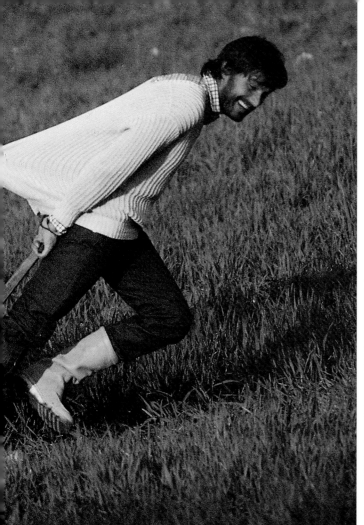

daily use, and the number is increasing every year. The toxic effects of 80 per cent of these substances are unknown. Yet synthetic chemicals are believed to cause up to ten per cent of all cancer deaths.

Toxic chemicals applied to farmland and sprayed into the air are building up in our food and water. Already over three million people in this country are drinking water with aluminium levels higher than is allowed by EEC regulations. Every day four million Britons drink water with excessive levels of nitrates, which are now thought to cause cancer.

The thinning of the world's ozone layer which protects us from the harmful side effects of the sun's ultraviolet rays is caused by gases from aerosol cans, refrigerators, and some hamburger cartons. In the USA alone scientists are predicting an increase of 40 million more skin cancers and 12 million eye cancers in the next 90 years.

More than 75 million acres of western Europe and North America have already been damaged by acid rain, and more than 150 acres of tropical rain forests are cut down every minute.

Our health depends upon a healthy, balanced planet earth. There are certain everyday products you can buy which have been known for some time to have a detrimental effect upon the environment – for instance, leaded petrol and aerosols containing chlorofluorocarbons. (CFCs). Avoid them.

If you are concerned about any of the products you are buying, check with your local green groups.

If you feel you have been overexposed to certain pollutants such as lead and aluminium, the effects may be counteracted by certain mineral supplements. (See POLLUTION.)

GREEN SHOPPING
Think twice before buying a product. Ask yourself:
Does it endanger your health and that of others?
Does it damage the environment during manufacture or disposal?
Does it use materials from threatened species or threatened environments?
Does it involve cruelty to animals, either in testing or for other reasons?
Does it consume a disproportionate amount of energy during manufacture, disposal or use?
Is it overpackaged, causing waste, or does it have an unduly short useful life?

the broadest part of your face.
● High bridges emphasise long noses.
● Tops of glasses should echo eyebrow shape as closely as possible.
● Check that glasses fit neatly over the nose without slipping.
● Long thin face? Choose frames with strong horizontal lines.
● Delicate frames strengthen petite features. Large frames make faces look smaller.
● A round face? Choose geometric shapes and avoid spindly frames.
● Heart-shaped or broad faces can wear winged or decorated frames.

Green

A healthy body and mind require a healthy environment. Much of the world's disease is caused by environmental pollution. Acid rain, polluted water and synthetic chemicals are all contributory factors.

Environmentalists are concerned about what are now termed green issues; they are concerned about the following facts. . . .

Over 70,000 chemicals are in

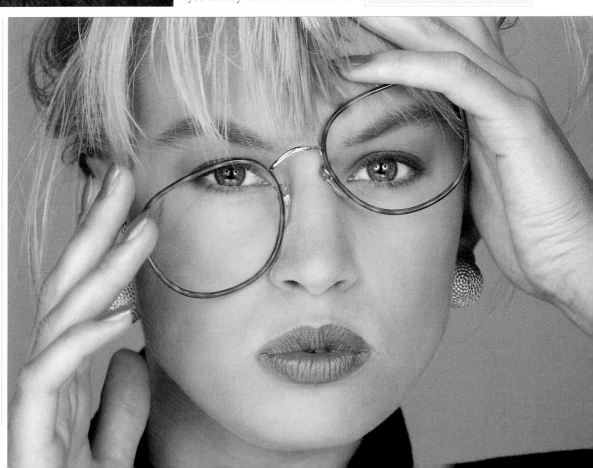

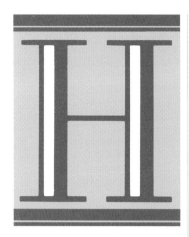

HAIR

Hair is composed mainly of a protein called keratin along with traces of mineral substances. Each hair consists of three layers: the spongy tissues of the central core or *medulla*; the cortex which consists of long thin cells that give hair its elasticity and colour; and the outer layer, known as the cuticle, which is made up of hundreds of tiny overlapping scales.

As hair is a dead substance, its condition depends upon a healthy scalp. Stimulate the circulation in your scalp with a vigorous massage for five minutes twice a day: plant the tips of all your fingers and thumbs firmly in a close pattern on one area of your scalp. Stretch the scalp in every direction, massaging it as vigorously as you can for a few seconds, then move on to another area. Also brush the hair thoroughly for three to five minutes each day.

FOOD FOR HAIR CARE

Every year we spend millions on products promising to thicken or straighten our hair, or make it shine. But nothing improves the condition of hair more effectively than a good, balanced diet containing all the essential minerals and vitamins that contribute to glossy, shining hair.

● Brittle, limp hair indicates an iron deficiency. Iron-rich foods include parsley, green vegetables, liver, eggs.
● Sulphur contributes to healthy hair – found in eggs, cabbage, dried beans, fish, nuts and meat.
● Zinc – helps prevent hair loss. Eat wheat bran, wheatgerm, turkey, lamb and eggs. (See ZINC.)
● B vitamins – essential for glossy colour and thickness. Deficiencies may lead to loss of colour and could encourage grey hair. Include brewer's yeast, liver, bananas and soya beans in your diet. (See VITAMINS.)

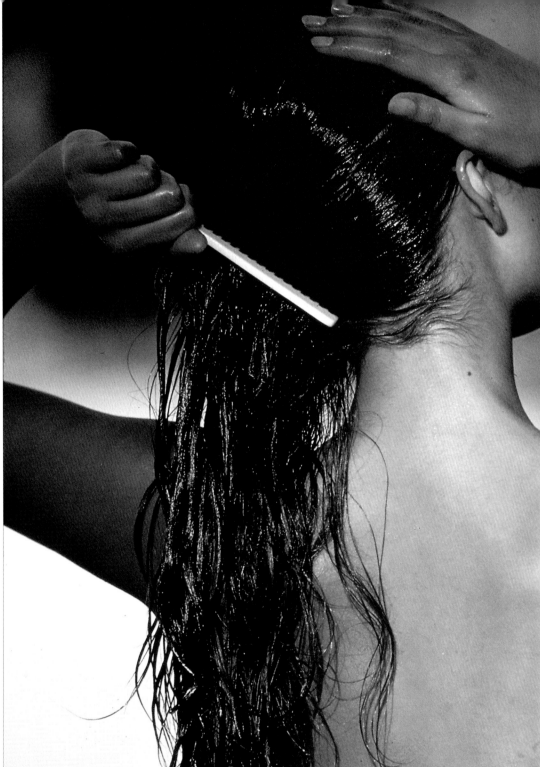

● Vitamin C – ensures the health of the capillaries supplying blood to hair follicles. Make sure your diet includes plenty of fresh fruit and vegetables.
● Vitamin E – encourages hair growth. Switch from refined flours to wholemeal and wheatgerm.

SHAMPOO

Once your diet is geared to shiny, healthy hair you can concentrate on selecting a suitable shampoo for your particular hair type. The cheaper shampoos usually include petroleum-based oils (as in washing-up liquids) and may also contain chemical foam boosters and foam stabilisers which can strip hair of its natural oils. Better quality shampoos are more likely to be found in health food shops and are unlikely to contain animal ingredients. Always use a conditioner after shampooing – it makes hair manageable. The longer you can give your hair a break between shampoos the better. Too frequent shampooing can tear some of the fibres of protein.

Leaving your hair to nature helps build up the scalp's natural cleansing oils. The following are good types of shampoo to try:
Balsam – a resin from the bark of certain trees. For fine hair that lacks body. It thickens and strengthens hair by coating the hair shaft.
Camomile – has mild bleaching properties so keeps blonde hair shiny.
Lemon – best for oily, fair hair. Restores hair's natural acid coating.

Protein – most protein shampoos contain protein from eggs, milk, beef or soya and lightly coat the outer layer of hair. Others, called substantive proteins, strengthen the follicle and are effective for treating fine hair that is damaged.

Rosemary – especially for dark hair. Refreshes scalp.

STYLING PRODUCTS

Gel – creates slick, structured styles. Can be used as a strong setting lotion for blow-drying curly hair straight.

Mousse – lightweight styling aid giving body and texture to hair. Best for fine hair, but don't apply when hair is dry – it will feel sticky. Wet hair dilutes the mousse. Towel dry hair and apply mousse, working through length of hair with hands.

Pomade/grease – contains wax. Use only a little to give sheen, control and hair separation. Best used on dark or black hair.

Shaping sprays, sculpting lotions – help mould style and give it staying power. Sprays can add body to the roots. Application varies: some can be used on wet hair, others on dry.

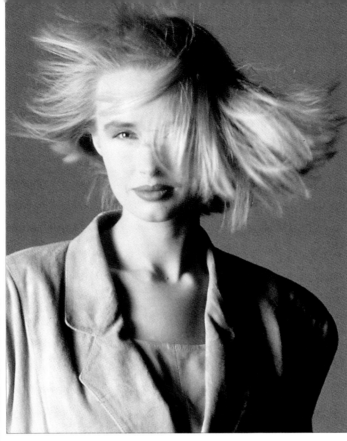

HAIR COLOUR

People often change their hair colour when they experience or desire a major change in their lives; it can play an important part in building a new image.

If you are not sure whether a change of colour will suit you, try out a temporary or vegetable colourant first. A drastic change of colour could mean alterations to your wardrobe.

Constant bleaching and dyeing can fill the weakened hair with colouring chemicals that prevent cuticle scales from closing up and leaves hair looking rough and dry.

HAIR COLOUR GUIDE

Temporary colourants:
For minor colour changes that are close to natural colour. Cannot lighten hair, and will wash out after one or two shampoos.

Semi-permanents:
Good for camouflaging sprinklings of grey hair and highlighting natural colour. Will not lighten or drastically change hair colour, and will fade after about six shampoos.

Vegetable dyes:
Camomile – great for sun-streaking blonde and light brown hair after several applications.

Henna – a plant colourant that gives black and brunette hair a radiant reddish glow. Mixed with indigo, henna can colour the hair various shades of brown and black. Some henna products can also be used on blonde hair to give richness and shine, without the red colouring.

Metallic dyes
Darken grey hair by depositing metal dyes, salts and various metals in the hair shaft. Hair will not perm well, and often becomes dull.

Bleaching
Hydrogen peroxide penetrates the hair shaft and oxidises the pigments. Bleaching is often used with other permanent tints.

Aniline or oxidation colourants
These colourants make up the step-by-step packages bought at chemists. They are permanent, but one in ten women is allergic to them.

BLACK/AFRO/ASIAN

Measure half a cup of olive oil into a jar with one cup of runny honey. Shake well until mixed. Leave for two days. Shake before using and rub into hair. Leave for 20 minutes. Rinse well and add an infusion of rosemary or sage to last rinse.

BRUNETTE

The juice from the green shells surrounding fresh walnuts enhances brown hair. Mix 20g of ground green walnut husks with 50cc water, 25g alum and 75g salad oil. Warm mixture until it has the required colour and apply to the hair. Add vinegar to rinsing water.

BLONDE

Camomile is great for keeping blonde hair golden and gleaming. Use in shampoos or make a lukewarm infusion – 10g per 100cc boiling water – and when cool rinse hair.

Lemon also highlights blonde hair. Mix its juice with beaten egg and a tablespoon of honey and use as conditioner. Or rub freshly squeezed juice into the hair before washing. Leave for five minutes. Be careful to avoid your eyes.

REDHEAD

Use henna as a conditioner to give hair bounce and highlight red and copper tones. Mix powder to a paste and leave on hair for ten minutes only.

Reddish-brown onion skins can also be used to burnish red hair. Boil 30g onion skins in 200 mls of water and filter off clear liquid. Add 5g glycerin. Apply daily until highlights glow. Not for oily hair.

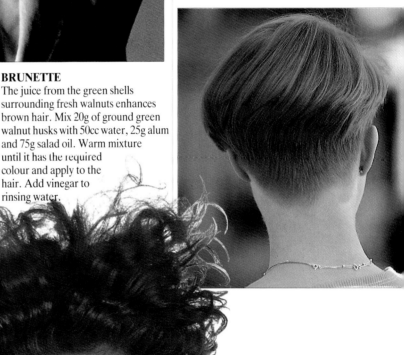

HAIR LOSS

Hair loss can be a problem for both men and women, and often causes distress.

Hair loss can be divided into four basic types: systematic – a reaction to medication, illness or hormone imbalance; hereditary – related to genes and there is very little you can do about it; infectious – a bacterial or fungal condition; and traumatic – damage to the scalp caused by excessive bleaching, perming, or colouring. Over 75 per cent of men over 40 show signs of balding but the process usually starts in the 20s with a receding hairline.

Men usually go bald because of a high level of male hormones which affects the functioning of the hair follicles. Hormones can also play a part in the hair loss experienced by women. Hair can start to fall out in handfuls when oestrogen levels drop around menopause. Hormone Replacement Therapy (see HRT) can help the condition. Pregnancy also causes hair loss, but the hair grows back to normal shortly after breastfeeding has ended. But there is little that can be done to reverse the balding experienced by men. It is usually hereditary. However, the process can be slowed by:

● Regular MASSAGE with a hair tonic.
● Preventing a build-up of stress which tightens muscles at the nape of the NECK and slows the circulation of blood to the scalp and follicles.
● A diet rich in nutrients needed for healthy hair growth. (See HAIR.)
● Nettles have always been thought to prevent hair loss. Chop 100g of nettles (the stinging kind!) and add to half a litre of boiling water. When cool, add half a litre of vinegar. Warm and use as a daily rinse for ten days.

HAIR TRANSPLANTS
Transplanting is an expensive and slow process. It involves grafting plugs of skin with eight or ten follicles. Approximately 100 grafts are needed to retrieve a receding hairline. It takes a while for the results to show – and generally gives a tufted, slightly unnatural appearance.

HAIR WEAVING
Used to cover a thinning patch. Hair is interwoven with Teflon threads creating a meshed base to which matching hair is attached.

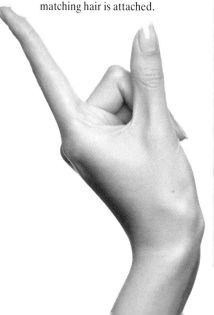

HANDS

Your hands have a hard life. They're exposed to all kinds of weather conditions, immersed in water containing powerful chemical solutions such as washing powder. No wonder they are the first parts of the body to show neglect and ageing.

Hands have relatively few oil glands compared with the rest of the body, so rub in hand cream as often as you can – especially after hands have been in water. Wear rubber gloves for household chores. Swap alkaline soaps for vegetable or glycerine-based ones which are less drying. Dry hands thoroughly afterwards.

If your hands have been neglected, start by rubbing off rough skin with a well-soaped pumice stone. Soak hands in a mixture of equal parts salt and Epsom salts dissolved in warm water to open pores and stimulate circulation. Dry and rub in hand cream.

Hands can get very tense – try a massage to release tension, stimulate circulation and improve skin tone. Apply three drops of benzoin, lavender, lemon or almond essential oil and massage into hands, working from wrists to palm and fingers as if easing out tension

---

NAIL FILE
Flaking, splitting, chipping
Moisturise daily with cuticle cream.
Use an oil-based lacquer remover. Wear rubber gloves for chores. Use nail hardener.
File nails in one direction only and don't shape into points.
Ridges
Indicates zinc or calcium deficiency, or damaged nail bed.
Use commercial ridge filler as a base before polish.
Hangnails
Caused by dry cuticles, biting and chewing.
Keep skin soft by daily moisturising.
Never pull or tear cuticle.
Yellowing
Caused by staining from orange and red nail varnish, pool chlorine, or smoking.
Use slough/buffer very lightly.
Soak nails in lemon juice.
White spots
Zinc deficiency or damage to nail bed.
Eat plenty of spinach, wholegrain products, sunflower seeds.

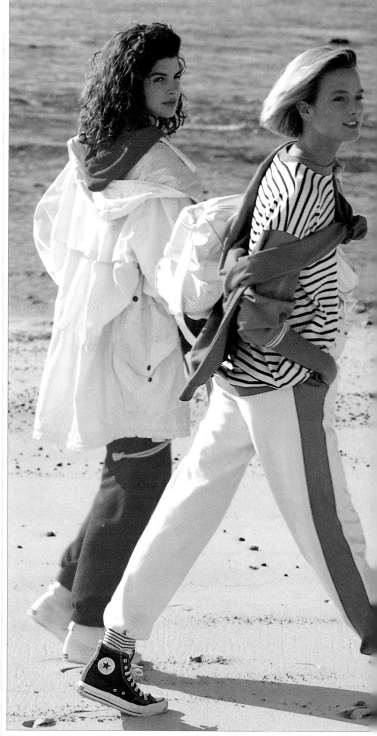

HEALTH

Health is not a destination in life but a way of travelling through it. Nor is health an absolute concept, but relative to an individual's own potential. Whether you are quick or slow, tall or short, prone to being thin or fat, or physically handicapped in some way, you have the capacity to achieve your full potential.

Realising this potential is not a question of reaching some measured idea of physical, mental, social and spiritual well-being. Neither is it simply a matter of following recommended guidelines on diet, exercise, and the balance of work, rest and play – although this is an excellent starting point!

Health is a state of harmony which can adapt to all the changes and influences in our environment and in ourselves. It is a simple transformation in your outlook on life – one which requires desire, will, discipline, common sense, adaptability and constant vigilance. It is the active process of caring for yourself, recognising your strengths

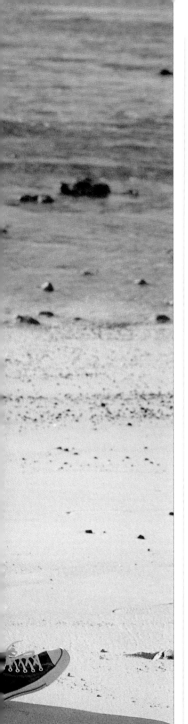

CHECK LIST		FREQUENCY OF TEST
BLOOD PRESSURE	30+	Every two years (Women taking the contraceptive pill every year.)
	50+	Every year
BREAST EXAMINATION		Examine breasts yourself every month. Doctor or family planning clinic should check every year. Mammograms should be done approximately every three years after 35
CERVICAL SMEAR	pre-35	Every two years
	35+	Every year
CHOLESTEROL	pre-35	Every three years
	35–50	Every two years
	50+	Every year
DENTAL		Every six months
EYESIGHT		Every year. Soft lens wearers every six months
GYNAECOLOGICAL EXAMINATION	pre-35	Every three years
	35–49	Every two years
	50+	Every year
HEART AND LUNGS		As for cholesterol
URINE		As for cholesterol

excellent method of screening as specific diagnosis and early treatment can be completely effective.

Checking BLOOD PRESSURE can be useful, as long as it is not done in isolation from previous pressure checks. Blood pressure levels can vary from person to person and so an isolated reading will not give very much information. If blood pressure is high, it is best to aim to reduce stress and adapt your behaviour associated with stress – poor diet, smoking or drinking alcohol.

As the importance of preventive medicine is recognised, an increasing range of health checks are becoming available both on the NHS and privately. Keep a record of your health checks and make sure you have them regularly.

HEALTH RESORTS

Escape to a health resort for a few days and come back feeling on top of the world!

Thinking about taking a few days off? Feeling burnt out? Traditional holidays don't always offer an ideal opportunity for rest. Travelling adds to stress, and it often seems that by the time you have to leave, you are only just beginning to feel the benefit.

A health resort offers an opportunity to pamper yourself and need not cost more than a holiday abroad. The old image of health resorts is one of lettuce leaf dinners and strenuous exercise regimes for people desperate to lose weight. All

types of people from all walks of life – not necessarily overweight – enjoy the relaxed atmosphere of today's health resorts. Massage, beauty and health treatments, fresh nutritious foods and extra rest are all wonderful ways to reward yourself. If you are keen to improve your overall health by making changes to your lifestyle, a health resort can be an excellent launching pad. Trained staff are on hand to give advice should you need it, and both the facilities and menus are powerful incentives for altering unhealthy lifestyle patterns.

HEART

The heart is the power-house of the body. The right-hand side pumps blood to the lungs, where it collects oxygen and is cleansed of carbon dioxide and other wastes. The left side pumps the freshly oxygenated blood around the body so that it reaches every cell. At its most efficient the heart pumps up to 5,000 gallons of blood a day around a vast network of arteries, veins and capillaries.

The Chinese believed the heart stored 'shen' – the consciousness – but Western tradition sees it as the home of the emotions. The heart readily responds to emotions – when angry its pulse quickens and blood pressure shoots up.

The heart keeps fit on a diet rich in minerals and low in fats, salt and sugar. It loves exercise as well as relaxation techniques that combat stress. Extra weight makes it overwork, and nicotine raises its beat and adds to the risk of blood clotting. (See EXERCISE, CARDIOVASCULAR, RELAXATION.)

HERBALISM

The main purpose of herbal remedies is to stimulate the body's own natural healing abilities by rebalancing and cleansing it.

Herbalism is the world's oldest method of treating ill health. The earliest known records of medicinal herbs are in northern China, dating back to 3,000BC. A knowledge of herbal remedies has been handed down from generation to generation in most societies throughout the world, and has survived for centuries.

The World Health Organisation has been encouraging a revival of traditional herbal medicine in developing countries, but in parts of America the professional practice

and resources so that you can enjoy life, feel well, respond to challenge, know your limits and reach your full potential.

HEALTH CHECKS

The most useful type of health checks are those which can be acted upon to prevent disease. For example, death from some cancers is preventable, provided that the cancer is found early enough. Cervical cytology is therefore an

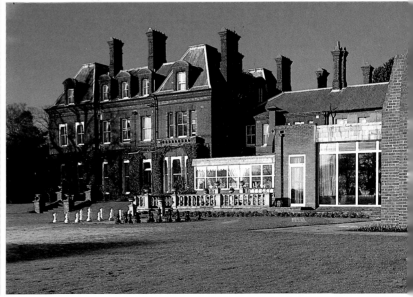

of herbalism is still illegal. In Britain herbalists are trained by the National Institute of Medical Herbalists and, unlike their predecessors of centuries ago, have a sophisticated understanding of the human body. The herbal approach is based on the assumption that an infection is a problem secondary to a lifestyle with which the sufferer's body cannot cope – possibly due to a dietary factor.

Herbal remedies are gentle and safe, and easy to use, but if in doubt consult a qualified herbalist. Use the plants and flowers growing in your garden or window boxes to create a herbal medicine chest of your own.

Pick plants on a dry morning when dew has evaporated. Choose only the healthiest specimens. Lay them out on a sheet of greaseproof paper as soon as possible in an airy room. Never dry herbs in the sun.

When stems can be used, such as with peppermint and sage, hang in small bunches from the ceiling in a well-aired room. Any mouldy plants should be thrown away.

After drying, store in a dark cupboard in airtight glass jars and label clearly.

You can now use them as infusions. (During pregnancy it is always advisable to seek professional advice before taking home remedies.)

For an infusion, steep herbs in boiling water for ten minutes. Strain and use.

For a standard infusion add 1oz (28g) of the dried herb to one pint of water but for a smaller amount add one to two teaspoons of dried herb to a cup of water.

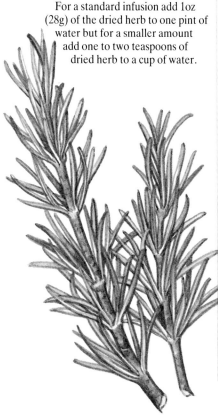

HERBAL INFUSIONS
Camomile – a gentle sedative, and can be taken as often as enjoyed

Elderflower – a diuretic. Helps body sweat out accumulated toxins. Take one cup three times a day

Marigold – excellent for skin problems such as eczema, minor burns and bruising. Can be used in a COMPRESS

Passion flower – for nervous conditions such as spasmodic asthma and insomnia. Drink one small cup daily

Rosemary – aids digestion and calms nervous tension. Take one cup three times a day

---

H**IPS**

Men tend to gather fat around their hips from the early 30s onwards – a warning that a POT BELLY is well on the way.

Women's hip are more flexible than men's because of their ability to bear children, and they naturally carry more fat deposits.

Men can improve their flexibility through YOGA, and stretching exercises. Cycling, swimming and dancing are all good for hip mobility.

Middle-age spread is *not* inevitable. Invest in a hula hoop and stop those pads of fat settling around the hips. It takes practice, but once mastered, swivelling movements will keep your waist in trim, too.

After a bath or shower, massage with a loofah, sisal mitt or soft body-brush. If fat is a problem, knead hips daily with a moisturising cream containing ivy extract.

H**IV**

TheHumanImmunodeficiency Virus (HIV) can cause AIDS and two milder Aids-related conditions – Aids Related Complex (ARC) and Persistent and Generalised Lymphadenopathy (PGL). HIV weakens the body's immune system by infecting a specific group of lymphocyte cells in the bloodstream. The lymphocytes are the main command and control centre of the immune system; when these cells are unable to function properly the immune system is no longer able to defend the body against infection.

Once infected with HIV, the body

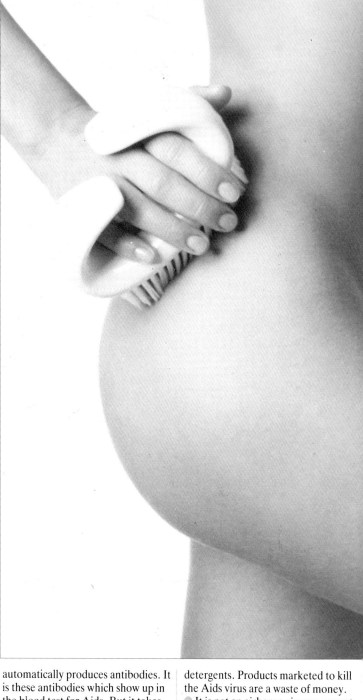

automatically produces antibodies. It is these antibodies which show up in the blood test for Aids. But it takes the body several weeks to produce antibodies to the HIV virus; during this 'window period' a person can be infected and infectious and still give a negative test result.   Experts say that most people who are diagnosed HIV antibody positive will probably go on to develop full-blown Aids within 15 years.

The HIV infection has been exploited by many people to support a variety of prejudices, especially against the gay community.

We do know:
● HIV is a fragile virus which survives only in body fluids and dies quickly outside the body. HIV is killed by heat, household bleach and detergents. Products marketed to kill the Aids virus are a waste of money.
● It is not an airborne virus so cannot be transmitted through coughs and sneezes.
● People can live with virus carriers without risk, sharing cups, plates, living space (but not razors or toothbrushes because of infection via broken skin and blood).
● You cannot catch HIV from towels, toilet seats or normal social contact.
● Men who have the virus give it to sexual partners through semen, blood or other body fluids entering the partner's body.
● Women who have the virus can give it to their sexual partners via vaginal secretions or exchange of other bodily fluids such as blood and urine, and to

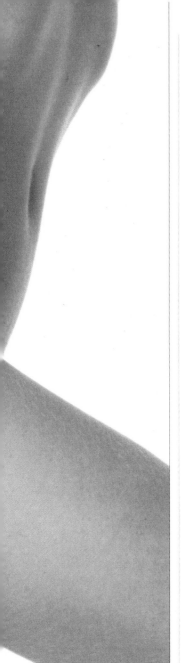

HOLISTIC MEDICINE

Holistic medicine is an overall term embracing an approach to illness by all practitioners of alternative therapies (eg OSTEOPATHY, AROMATHERAPY, ACUPUNCTURE).

Holistic diagnosis and treatment take into account body, mind and spirit as well as environmental factors. Symptoms of ill health are never isolated from a patient's general and mental health. A holistic approach to ill health can involve several therapies to treat one particular ailment – often complementary to orthodox medicine.

HOMOEOPATHY

Homoeopathy is based on the principle 'curing like with like' and is unique among the alternative therapies in that it is available on the National Health Service.

Samuel Hannemann, a German doctor, discovered in the first half of the 19th century that the symptoms produced by quinine in a healthy body were remarkably similar to the symptoms which quinine was used to treat. He also developed 'potentisation' – the use of tiny doses of a particular drug to produce a more powerful effect.

Homoeopathy regards the symptoms of disease as part of the body's attempt to defend itself from illness, so diagnosis is based on symptoms rather than causes.

Most homoeopathic medicines are prepared from fresh plant and animal sources. They are prescribed only after the homoeopath has drawn up a comprehensive picture of the patient's mental and emotional state, diet etc. The remedy that produces symptoms closest to those of the individual will be curative.

Homoeopathic medicines are safe for everyone including children, pregnant women and the elderly.

HONEY

Ancient Greeks considered honey to be the food of the gods and for centuries its healing properties have been recognised.

Honey is easy to digest, and contains mineral salts and formic acid – the bee's own chemical additive which gives it its antiseptic qualities and prevents spoilage. It also contains

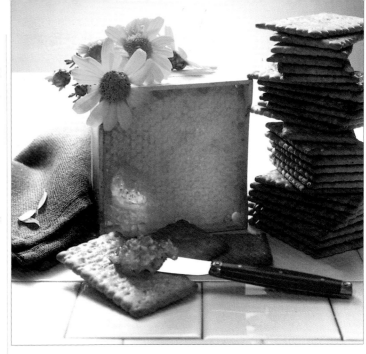

the properties of the flowers the bees have been browsing among. Linden honey, for example, will be calming, while rosemary will be stimulating.

Added to warm water, honey will soothe a sore throat or tonsillitis but apart from its medicinal qualities, it is an essential beauty aid. It can be used on its own as a face mask for dry or normal skin, or combined with oatmeal to refine greasy skin.

It makes an excellent hair conditioner – add a tablespoon of honey and two teaspoonfuls of vegetable oil to a beaten egg. Massage into hair and leave for half an hour before shampooing.

Use instead of sugar whenever you can, but if taken in large quantities honey can cause tooth decay and act as a laxative.

HORMONES

Hormones influence the functioning of the body's systems and organs and are circulated through the bloodstream by the endocrine glands. The glands control a variety of the body's functions – for instance, the adrenal glands are involved in a variety of body functions including the metabolism of starches and response to stress, the parathyroid glands regulate the levels of calcium, the ovaries and testes produce the male and female hormones and regulate the reproductive cycle and lactation.

The endocrine network is regulated by the pituitary gland situated below the brain. Other endocrine glands include the thyroid and pancreas.

HRT
(HORMONE REPLACEMENT THERAPY)

During MENOPAUSE, the female hormones oestrogen and progesterone dwindle. This affects women in a number of ways. They can experience menopausal side effects such as hot flushes, vaginal dryness, depression, irritability, OSTEOPOROSIS. Hormone replacement therapy (HRT) artificially reintroduces the missing hormones back into the body, alleviating the symptoms.

The treatment consists of a low dose of both hormones given in sequence mimicking menstrual cycle – the first two weeks take oestrogen only, the third week progesterone only and the last week nothing. Before taking HRT your blood should be tested to determine the level of hormones needed, and there should be at least three follow-up visits to ensure the balance is right. The treatment is taken in pill form, patches like plasters on the skin, or implants under the skin.

HRT FACT FILE
Take the lowest possible dose that will relieve symptoms. Once symptoms lessen decrease dosage.

HRT is only advisable for women whose symptoms are severe. Women suffering from diabetes, high blood pressure, clotting disorders, fibroids, phlebitis, breast cancer, heart and kidney complaints should make their condition known to their doctor when discussing HRT.

Contrary to popular belief, replacing oestrogen lost by the body will not make you look younger.

---

their babies through the placenta, or through breast milk.

Only a very small number of people have contracted HIV through blood transfusions, mostly before blood was being screened. All donors, donated blood and donated blood products are now screened.

In this country there is no danger of contracting the virus through donating blood or medical injections as disposable needles and syringes are used. This could be a problem in the Third World and you may want to take needles and syringes with you if you are travelling to a country with a shortage of medical equipment.

Intravenous drug users should not share needles and syringes.

It is practically impossible to catch the virus if you practise SAFE SEX.

● HRT does not delay menopause. It masks it. If you start HRT before your natural periods have stopped, bleeding will continue after you have reached the menopause.

● Fertility will not be affected in any way. You cannot have children once you have passed your natural menopause, whether or not you continue to bleed on HRT. A blood test will show whether you need to continue with contraception.

● HRT is not a contraceptive. You are still fertile and will continue to need contraception until your doctors says it is no longer necessary. (See MENOPAUSE.) You will not be able to take the contraceptive pill while you are having HRT.

● HRT has been associated with breast cancer, so have a breast examination every six months.

Interested? Contact your local Well Woman Clinic, Family Planning Clinic or doctor.

HYDROTHERAPY

The healing properties of natural hot and cold water springs were recognised by many ancient civilisations, but it was not until the 16th century that water 'cures' were developed in Europe around mineral springs and wells, so creating spa towns. Today, hydrotherapy includes the use of water internally and externally in the form of baths, packs, compresses, sprays, and special exercises performed in pleasantly warm, therapeutic pools.

The natural buoyancy of the water allows a wider range of movement and is especially suitable for the physically handicapped. Other hydrotherapy practices include whirlpools, steam treatments and saunas.

Hydrotherapy is most frequently prescribed for patients suffering from musculoskeletal or neurological disorders. If you are recommended hydrotherapy by your doctor, treatment will usually be given in the therapeutic pool of the nearest hospital or local spa. The pool will be small and very warm and the water will come up to the waist. The therapist will show you exercises to strengthen weak and damaged muscles and loosen stiff joints.

The hydrotherapist may also recommend the application of alternate hot and cold water to specific parts of your body in the form of baths, packs or special COMPRESSES.

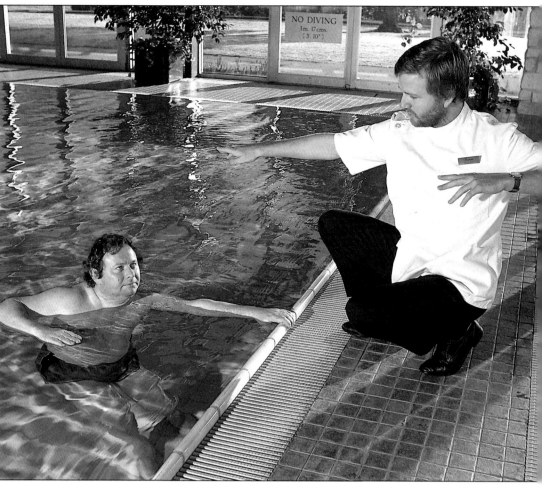

Many European spas became famous for their waters, including Malvern in England, Vichy in France and Marienbad in Czechoslovakia. Different treatments are offered including thalassotherapy (salt water treatments) and the Kneipp water cure based on lots of fresh air, regular exercise and water.

HYPERTENSION
(HIGH BLOOD PRESSURE)

It is normal for the pressure of the blood pumped out of the heart to increase during exertion and emotional stress.

In a healthy body it will return to normal quite quickly but continued high blood pressure places an extra strain on the heart and the kidneys and can lead to a stroke or coronary thrombosis.

Stress, lack of exercise, excess weight and hereditary factors can all cause high blood pressure.
To avoid high blood pressure you should remember the following pointers:
● Exercise
● Learn to relax
● Keep weight down
● Don't smoke
● Give up coffee, tea, chocolate
● Reduce sugar intake
● Reduce salt
● Shut out disturbing noises
● Talk more slowly!
(See MASSAGE, SMOKING, EMOTIONS, EXERCISE, AEROBICS.)

HYPNOTHERAPY

Hypnosis channels the resources of the unconscious to effect therapeutic change.

When someone is in a hypnotic trance, the conscious mind is sufficiently relaxed for the therapist to communicate suggestions to the subject's unconscious mind. Hypnotherapy and self-hypnosis help with high blood pressure, asthma, migraine, skin diseases, ulcers, stress, depression and anxiety, and can also help control stammering, overeating and smoking.

A patient is put into a trance either by direct means – for example with a bright light, pendulum, metronome or the hypnotherapist's voice – or by the use of subtle, indirect suggestions and stories that carry a special meaning for the patient.

When you are successfully hypnotised, the therapist will use aspects of your mind as sources of guidance to your present problem. For instance, the therapist may draw on childhood feelings of energy and good health to help combat constant, unexplained tiredness.

HYPOTENSION
(LOW BLOOD PRESSURE)

Low blood pressure is generally a positive health advantage – it shows the heart is not under considerable strain and indicates the body has a far greater degree of reserve for emergencies.

A major indication of problematic low blood pressure is when faintness or giddiness follow a sudden change of movement from sitting to standing, or lying to sitting. Blood pressure soon returns to normal.

Low blood pressure only becomes a serious problem after sudden and extreme loss of body fluids during surgery, after haemorrhaging or prolonged bouts of vomiting.

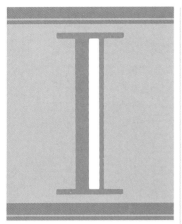

IMMUNE SYSTEM

The body's ability to resist infection – its immune system – depends on the power of certain white cells to distinguish friend from foe. Killer white cells, called phagocytes, roam the body destroying alien organisms (antigens) in the blood. If this first line of attack fails, B lymphocytes take over and make specially tailored antibodies which surround and destroy the antigen. Equally vigilant are T lymphocytes which kill invaders, or cancer cells, by producing hormone-like substances called lymphokines.

Lymphocytes reach all the tissues via the body's network of lymph channels. (See LYMPHATIC SYSTEM.) The battle of alien versus lymphocyte produces strong reactions, including rashes, swollen glands and fever, which are all part of the body's self-healing process.

Lymphocytes also have the ability to remember a particular invader and create immunity to it – which is why you normally don't get measles twice.

There are many things we don't know about the immune system, although the recent discovery of the HIV virus which gradually breaks down the immune system means it is now being studied intensively. Recent research is confirming what was always suspected – poor diet, negative thinking and stress can weaken the immune system's ability to fight for us. To stay healthy, we need to keep our immune system strong.

Foods for immunity

One of the most vital vitamins for the immune system is vitamin C. So eat plenty of fresh fruit – especially citrus fruits and leafy and green vegetables such as brussels sprouts, cabbage,

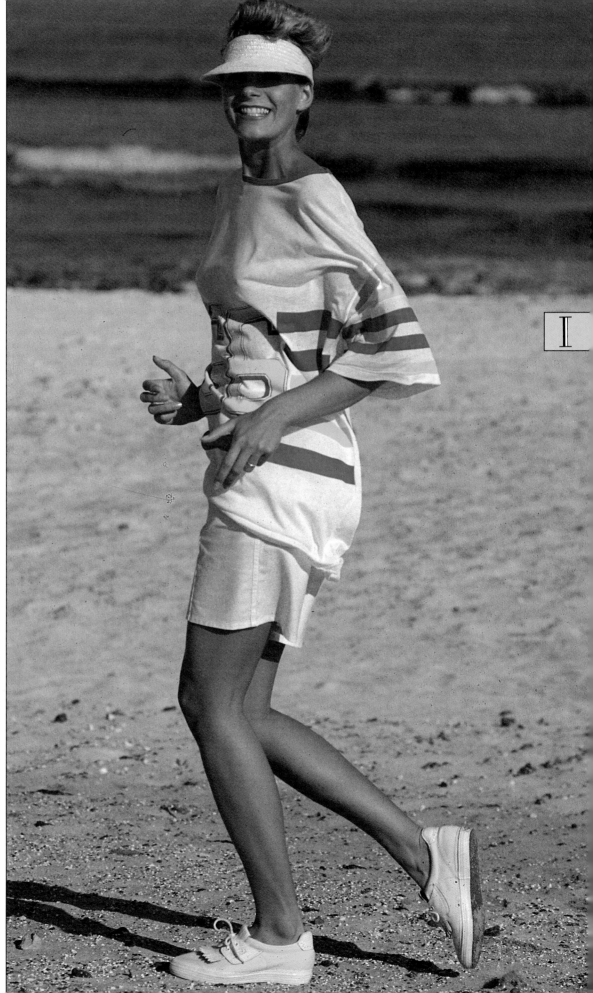

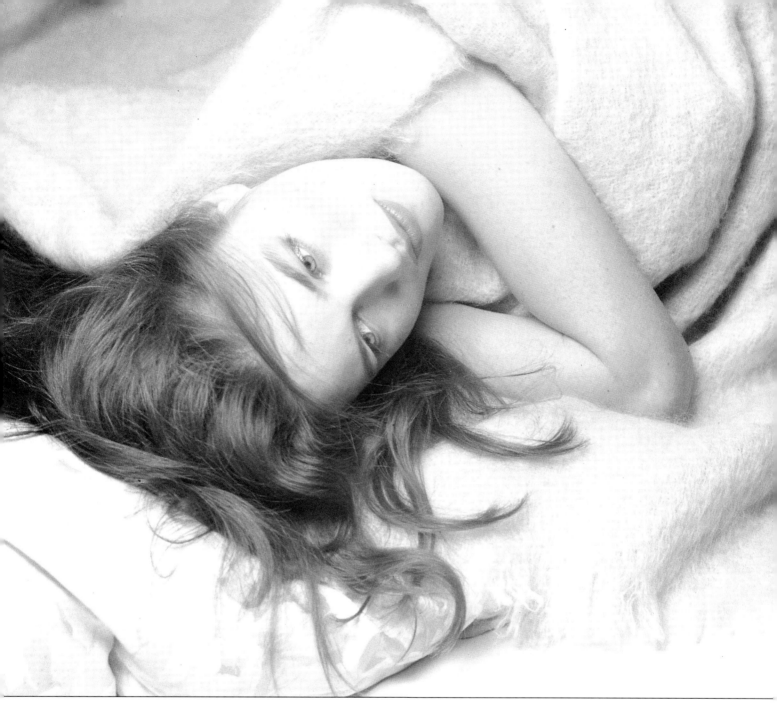

spinach and broccoli. Vitamin C cannot be stored in the body, so intake needs to be daily. Smoking destroys vitamin C; if you smoke, take supplements.

● Selenium protects the body tissues and enhances primary and secondary immune defences. Found in milk, eggs, fish, wholegrain cereals and meat.

● Zinc is important for fighting viral attacks. Found in fish, poultry, red meat, eggs, milk, dairy products and wholegrain cereals.

● Boost your immune system by eating plenty of raw foods – highly processed food robs the body of essential nutrients and weakens the immune system. Steam or gently

stir fry vegetables.

● Don't overeat. Recent studies show that a low-calorie, high-nutrition diet, with plenty of the above foods, delays the natural degeneration of the immune system.

Mind over matter
When we're overstressed, depressed, lonely or just feeling low, our immune system is affected too – leaving us vulnerable to all kinds of illness. There are ways you can think yourself healthier. POSITIVE THINKING wards off infection by boosting natural immunities…

● Block negative thoughts before they start – always think of at least one positive thing about a person or

situation you don't like.

● Give yourself a treat every day. It doesn't have to be expensive – an hour watching the television, a relaxing, scented bath, a walk through the park.

● Don't bottle up feelings. (See EMOTIONS.)

● Picture yourself feeling better – feed positive imagery into your mind. Some cancer patients have shown that by picturing the white cells actually destroying the invaders they could boost production of lymphocytes.

● Saying no to STRESS is another immune system booster.

● Learn relaxation techniques and don't overcrowd your life.

● Learn to delegate.

● Exercise regularly. (See AEROBICS, EXERCISE, FITNESS.)

INSOMNIA

Insomnia is rarely a permanent condition. It tends to coincide with periods of stress, anxiety, depression or other emotional disturbances. Once sleep patterns are disturbed, they are often extremely difficult to re-establish. For some people, the worry that they are not sleeping actually causes insomnia. People tend to need less sleep as they grow older and many people need only as little as four hours a

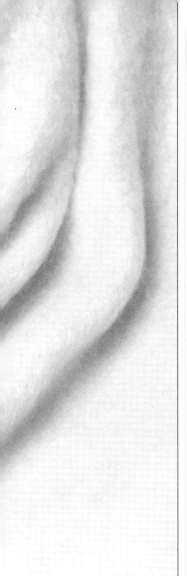

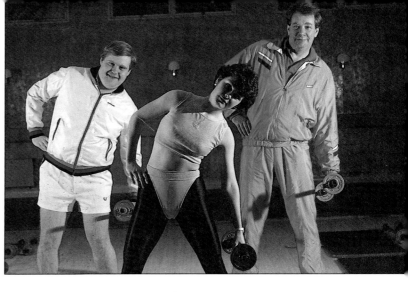

technique during the day. It will help you cope with stress and tension. (See RELAXATION, MEDITATION.)

● Get your partner to give you a soothing all-over MASSAGE.

ONS

Air ions are negatively and positively charged particles found in the air. They affect levels of a substance called serotin which is believed to have a calming effect upon the body. The full benefit of negative ions is best felt by the sea and in the mountains where they are abundant.

Positive ions are produced by air conditioning, central heating, tobacco smoke and electrical equipment and create feelings of lethargy and depression. Counter this effect with an ioniser to produce negative ions. Use one on your desk, by your bed or in your car.

RIDOLOGY

It was an owl that led to the development of iridology – the diagnosis of physical and mental disorders by studying the iris of the eye. In the 19th century Ignatz von Peczely, a Prussian surgeon, noticed that his pet owl's irises changed when its leg was fractured – the leg healed and marks on the irises disappeared.

Peczely then noted similar changes in the eyes of his patients and discovered that each mark in a different area of the iris corresponded with a particular part of the body. He divided both irises into a large number of 'reflex' areas. Iridology is now widely used by naturopaths and other therapists. In Australia iridology is used alongside orthodox medicine.

RON

Iron is needed by the body to produce haemoglobin – the transporter of oxygen around the body. It also strengthens the hair and nails.

Sixty per cent of British women between the ages of 18 and 54 do not get enough iron and are anaemic. The typical symptoms of anaemia are fatigue, breathlessness, headaches, loss of appetite, and palpitations.

The most common cause of anaemia is a diet deficient in iron,

vitamin B12 and vitamin C. Eggs, leafy green vegetables, potatoes, seafood, whole grains, parsley, watercress and liver all contain iron. Vitamin C aids its absorption. Iron is easily lost in cooking, so save your vegetable cooking water for soups and gravies. Better still, steam all vegetables.

SOMETRICS

An exercise method that strengthens, shapes and tones the body without moving strenuously. The advantage of isometrics is that it can be done anywhere at any time – in the home, at the office, in the train, waiting for a kettle to boil or lying in bed. Isometrics are based on the principle that you push or pull against objects that are immovable.

Isometric exercises can profitably while away irritating delays. For instance, while waiting for someone to answer the phone try this exercise to strengthen arms, shoulders and back . . .

Hold the receiver to your ear with one hand and with your free hand try to push down the nearest wall. Push as hard as you can with your

palm. Repeat with the other arm.

Waiting at the traffic lights in your car? Work on your abdominal muscles. Keep hands on the steering wheel, arms straight, sit erect, exhale fully, then tighten the abdominal muscles. For the back muscles, grip the steering wheel, straighten your arms and push back as hard as you can against the seat.

● Isometrics do not promote overall fitness and are not advisable for people with heart disease.

SOTONICS

Isotonic exercise, such as weight lifting and yoga, involves movement of the joints to achieve the rhythmic lengthening and shortening of muscles.

This type of exercise strengthens and tones muscles and adds grace and suppleness to the body's movements.

Ideally an exercise programme should combine isotonics with aerobics. For example, combine 15 minutes of stretching exercises with your favourite daily aerobic activity. (See AEROBICS, STRETCHING.)

I

day. High achievers seem to need less than the average eight hours.

To re-establish normal sleeping patterns avoid sleeping pills – they are physically and psychologically addictive. Instead of tossing and turning in bed worrying about not sleeping, get busy...

● Write letters, clean the bathroom, read a book, watch a late-night movie until you start to feel tired.

● Have a warm bath.

● Don't exercise before sleep – it stimulates rather than sedates.

● Sip camomile or lime blossom tea to relax. (See HERBALISM.)

● Avoid heavy meals and stimulants before bedtime.

● Practise a meditation or relaxation

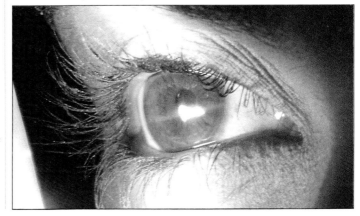

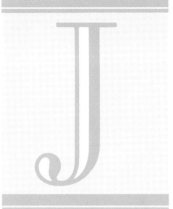

JET LAG

Jet lag is the end result of being hurtled through four time zones or more at a speed of over 450 mph for more than four hours.

You may arrive at your destination confused, exhausted and depressed; you can't settle into a routine – your appetite doesn't coincide with local meal times, you want to sleep at the 'wrong' time, you get constipated and there may be disturbing mood swings. Travelling east will double the effect of travelling west. Heading north or south seems to produce fewer symptoms of jet lag.

BEAT THE JET LAG BLUES
Setting off
⚪ Try to make time for some exercise before the flight.
⚪ Don't eat heavy meals or drink alcohol; eat only light foods, including lots of salad and fruit if possible.

You're flying
⚪ Drink lots of water and/or fruit juices. No alcohol or smoking. (See FLYING.)
⚪ Move around as much as possible.

You've landed
⚪ If you have to go into immediate action on arrival, eat a high protein meal (eggs, cheese, yoghurt, pulses, fish and nuts) at the normal breakfast time for your new base. Eat a high carbohydrate dinner (pasta, potatoes, whole grains) several hours before bedtime.
⚪ Don't catnap during the day.
⚪ You may not feel like it, but studies show that physical activity, such as a walk or swim after landing can reduce jet lag. Bright light also appears to help, so spend as much time in daylight as you can.

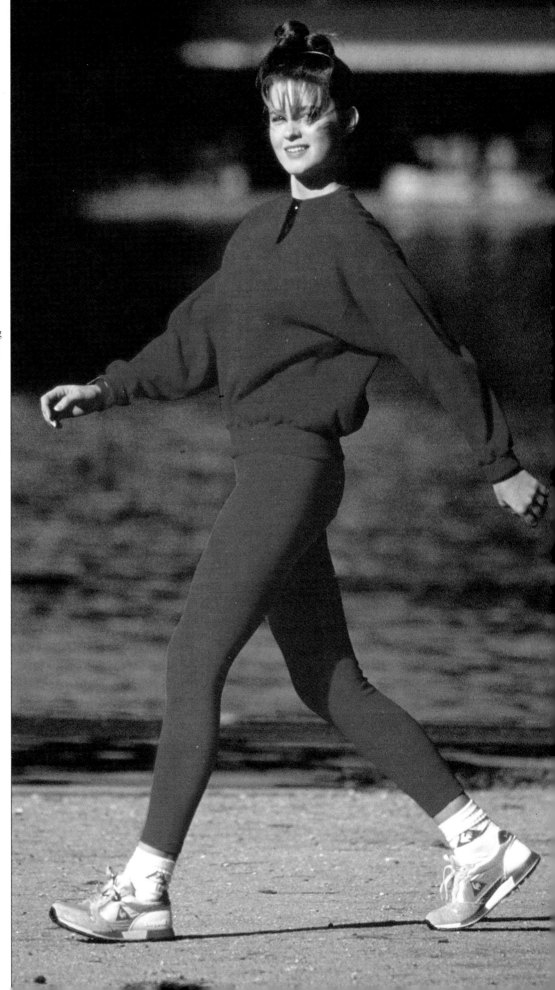

JOJOBA

Jojoba is a gentle, non-irritant oil used in both the cosmetic and manufacturing industries. It makes an excellent moisturiser, as it is easily absorbed into the skin and also helps improve the condition of the hair and scalp.

It is also used for coating pills and as a lubricant in open heart surgery.

The jojoba plant grows in most hot, arid areas and for centuries people of the desert have been using the oil from its beans to treat their hair and skin. The plant takes ten years to reach maturity and then produces ten pounds of beans each year for about 100 years. Jojoba oil is unlike any other animal or vegetable oil: it is non-toxic, does not go rancid, needs no chemical refinements and remains chemically unchanged for many years.

JUNK FOOD

Most pre-packaged, pre-cooked fast foods contain chemical additives, refined flours and sugars. Cream cakes, chocolate bars and soft drinks are all junk foods, too, and *addictive*.

A busy lifestyle means that an occasional fast-food meal or takeaway is inevitable, but problems arise when they become the main source of nourishment or you are only snacking on chocolate and crisps.

Need to cut down on excessive junk food consumption? Here's how:

You don't have to promise yourself, 'From Monday I am never going to eat junk food again.' The chances are that by Friday you'll be tucking into a fast hamburger for lunch and feeling horribly guilty and depressed by it. Instead launch yourself into an exercise care programme with regular AEROBICS, pamper your body with moisturisers and drops of aromatic oils in your baths, have a new hairdo, overhaul your DIET, and eat plenty of fresh fruit and vegetables. After three months of this regime, your desire for junk foods will disappear.
- Replace junk foods with wholemeal snacks like pasta, noodles, crackers and brown rice.
- Replace sweet milk shakes, ice cream and ice lollies with fresh fruit sorbets and yoghurt drinks.
- Reduce the junk element of your meal. Have that fast burger in a wholemeal bun. Order wholemeal chappattis instead of fried paratha.
- Substitute products such as crisps with dried fruits and unsalted nuts, carrot sticks.
- Wholemeal rolls and sandwiches make great snacks. Fill them with cottage cheese, beansprouts, lettuce and tomato, chopped liver, egg and spinach.

Your body will reward you once you've kicked the junk habit in favour of healthy wholesome foods. Eyes and hair will shine, muscles will firm, skin will clear and you'll feel revitalised.

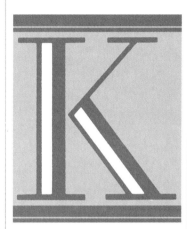

KEGEL EXERCISE

A woman's pelvic floor is made up of sheets of muscles suspended between the womb (uterus) from the pubic bone at the front and the tailbone at the back. They support the uterus, vagina, bladder and bowel. You can locate the muscles by trying to slow down or stop the flow of urine. Your ability to control the flow is an indication of how strong your muscles are.

Surgeon Arnold Kegel at the University of California has devised a series of exercises that are now standard practice for women after childbirth, and are ideal for toning vaginal muscles and holding everything else in place. They're great for improving sex and insure against prolapsed uterus.

Think of your pelvic floor as a slow lift and your normal state as the first floor. Slowly tighten the muscles, imagining the lift moving up to the second floor. Then tighten a little more and more to the third floor, and on to the fourth. Now, relax slightly, making stops at the third floor, second floor and finally the first. Then go down to the basement – your muscles will bulge out a little. Do five Kegels at least ten times a day. You can do them anywhere, and no one except you will ever know!

KELP

Kelp is a seaweed that grows in mineral-rich seawater. It contains vitamins B, D, and K and strengthens hair and nails. It is believed to control obesity and is sometimes used to treat ulcers and chronic constipation.

Kelp should not be taken by women planning pregnancy or pregnant, and, as no safe dosage has yet been established, it is wise not to take kelp over long periods.

KIDNEYS

The kidneys are among the hardest workers in the body. Without them we would be poisoned by our own wastes. We have two kidneys, one at each side of the backbone between the thick muscles of the back and abdomen. They are bean-shaped and about the size of a cupped hand.

They service all circulating blood every five minutes, clearing toxins and wastes through their tiny filters (nephrons) and excreting them from the body in urine. They control the balance of potassium and sodium in the blood, help in the production of red cells and regulate blood pressure.

If any of these functions break down, the build up of poisons in the body can become life-threatening.

For the Chinese the kidneys are 'the roots of life' and store 'jing' the substance of organic life.

Here's how to keep them healthy…
- Eat plenty of raw fresh foods and fibre. (See DIET.)
- Avoid foods with hidden toxins – additives, factory farmed or sprayed products – if you can. (See GREEN.)
- Drink plenty of fluids – preferably WATER, herb teas and juices – four pints a day is recommended.
- Cut down on salt.

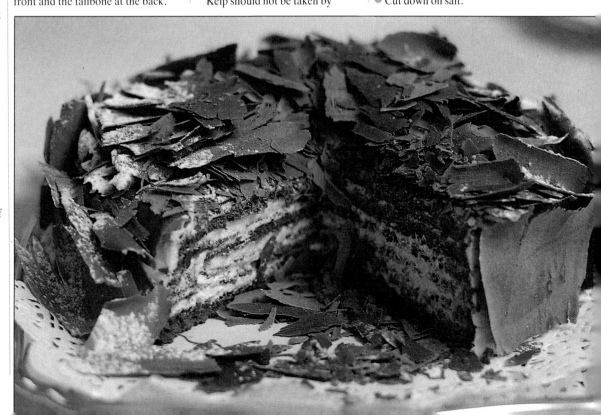

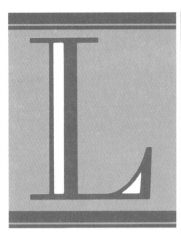

LAUGHTER

Laughter is not only a powerful antidote to stress, but studies have also shown that the more we laugh, the longer we live and the less prone we are to viral infections – especially if we have a loving partner to share our laughter with.

Laughter really is the best medicine… it's used to help adult aphasics regain speech and to treat autistic children with phobias, as well as anxiety in children. Laughter therapy is increasingly being used to overcome depression. It has cosmetic value too – the more you laugh the fewer your wrinkles.

Like good sex, laughing leaves you feeling relaxed and with a wonderful sense of well-being and security. When we laugh our hearts beat faster, adrenaline production increases, and the brain secretes natural opiate-like substances which find their way into the tears we shed and make us feel on a 'high' while laughing.

The saying 'Laugh and the world laughs with you, weep and you weep alone' has a ring of truth. People laugh more often when they are in groups – the more crowded a room, the greater the laughter – possibly to reduce the tension that results from overcrowding, or is it because laughter is infectious?

What makes us laugh? Psychological research has show seven main classes of ticklers: triumph, surprise, tickling, funny stories, incongruous situations, feeling happy, and as a cover for shyness. In the health stakes, laughter is certainly an essential daily ingredient, so enjoy it when you can.

If you're feeling down, concentrate on recalling an incident which has made you laugh… it won't be long before you're chuckling to yourself and the world seems a brighter place.

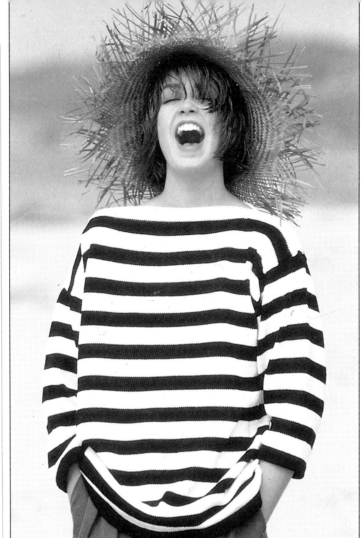

LEGS

In strict anatomical terms the leg is the part of the lower limb between the knee and the ankle, as distinct from the thigh. The skeleton of the leg is the tibia, which carries the body's weight, and the slender fibula alongside. Generally when people refer to the leg they include the thigh, too.

Extra weight, inactivity and a poor diet are the three major enemies of strong supple legs. They can cause varicose veins, impair circulation, thicken calves and swell ankles.

A balanced diet of natural unrefined foods discourages varicose veins and promotes free flow of blood to and from the legs. Plenty of exercise gets the circulation going and tones muscles; swimming is excellent for long leg muscles and cycling builds up leg power.

For those aching legs try BATHING in warm water with a few drops of clary sage, camomile or rosemary. Massage legs with warm olive oil and three drops of marjoram. Wrap with warm towels, rest for five minutes and

shower oil off with warm water. Rub skin with sea salt and rinse with cold water. Rub vigorously to dry, then gently massage with moisturiser.

Skiing is a sport which needs strong legs. The following exercises are used regularly by skiers to keep muscles strong and maintain stamina. So try this pre-ski workout every other day to firm and strengthen legs.

● *Full squat:* stand with legs shoulder width apart, lower buttocks until they are in line with knees (but not lower than the knees) and hold the position for eight seconds. Ensure knees are over toes, and heels are in contact with the floor. Repeat five times. Works thighs and calves.

● *Calf toner:* stand with arms straight out in front, legs straight, feet straight and together. Rise up on toes. Hold the position for eight seconds and then lower. Repeat eight times. Keep feet flat on the floor, bend forward at the knees eight times, repeat five times.

● *Inner thigh toner:* lie on one side, propped up by elbow, bottom leg straight, top leg bent over thigh of bottom leg with whole foot the floor. Hold stomach in and slowly

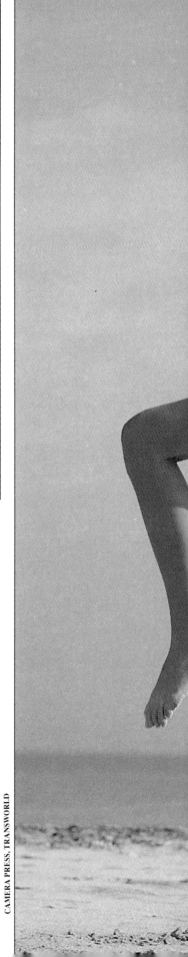

CAMERA PRESS, TRANSWORLD

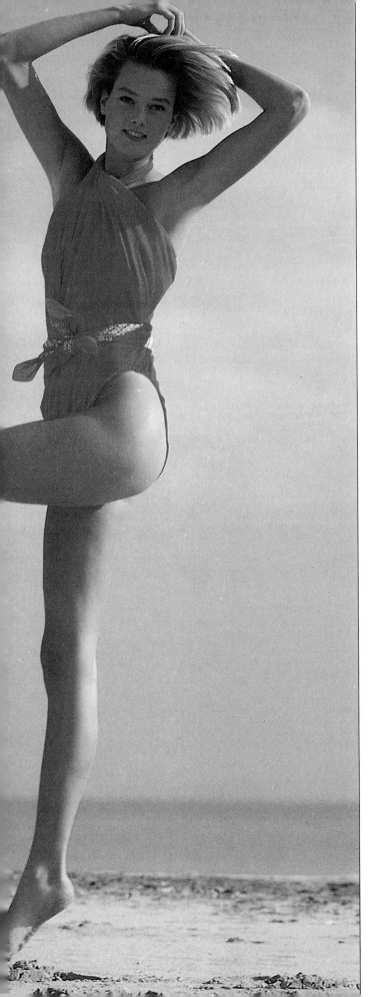

lift and lower bottom leg five times. Repeat 16 quicker repetitions at the top of each movement. Repeat on the other side.

LIPS

Unlike the rest of your skin, the lips contain no sebaceous glands to provide moisture and prevent cracking, or melanin to protect against the sun's ultra-violet rays. Lips easily become dehydrated and are vulnerable to extremes of weather. They need protecting…
● Coloured opaque zinc oxides protect lips against strong UV rays.
● When skiing choose an oily sunscreen to seal in moisture.
● If lips become chapped, don't pull skin – this can cause infection.
● Choose a soothing and repairing product to stimulate circulation and encourage faster healing.
● Waxy balms are best for keeping lips moist.

LIVER SPOTS

Generally known as age spots, these small brown blotches, like moles, appear on the back of the hands. Despite their names, they are not caused by age or the liver. They are a reaction to the sun's ULTRAVIOLET RAYS and there is very little that can be done about them. Avoid skin-bleaching agents, but try the following natural lotions – used over a period of time they should lighten the spots' dark pigment…
● Mix equal parts of lemon juice and rosewater, or cider vinegar, distilled water and milk. Leave on the skin for up to four hours. Wash off with warm tepid water, pat dry and apply an astringent followed by a rich moisturising cream.
If liver spots bother you, they can be professionally removed with liquid nitrogen or by skin peeling.

LUNGS

When we breathe in, air passes through our nose and into the lungs. The two primary bronchi which first bring the air into the lungs divide into smaller passages, which divide and subdivide into tubes that get smaller and smaller until they become tiny bronchioles To look at, the lungs are like an upside down tree in winter with the trachea forming the trunk, the primary bronchi the two main branches, and the bronchioles a network of smaller branches.

Healthy adult lungs can hold about five litres of air – nine milk bottles full. But we normally breathe only a fraction of that. Every living cell needs to combine food and oxygen to release energy. They receive this from a super-efficient supply system – blood.

The oxygen we breathe passes directly through the walls of minute air sacs – the alveoli – in the lungs into the blood stream. Waste carbon dioxide leaves the bloodstream in exactly the same way, eventually to be breathed out.

The lungs also filter out air dust and other particles in the atmosphere.

The total area of lung tissue reduces as you get older. In their prime, total lung surface measures roughly 100 square metres – as much as a wall-to-wall carpet in an average bedroom.

To help your lungs work efficiently and stay healthy, you can . . .
● Give up SMOKING.
● Take up regular exercise. Any aerobic exercise will get the lungs fit and in working order.
● Take supplements of anti-oxidant vitamins C and E to combat any over-exposure to air pollutants such as ozone, tobacco smoke, and formaldehyde (emitted from a chemical binding agent used to make building materials such as plywood). Make sure these VITAMINS along with vitamin A are included in your diet.
● Learn correct BREATHING. It keeps lungs in good working order and chest muscles and diaphragm strong.

LYMPHATIC SYSTEM

The lymphatic system is a network of lymph nodes spread around the body and connected by an intricate system of thin-walled channels that run throughout the body next to arteries and veins. The whole system is filled with a fluid called lymph – usually colourless and containing proteins, fats, lymphocytes and other substances. The nodes are found mainly in the neck, armpits, groin, behind the knees and around the heart.

The lymphatics return leaking serum protein to the bloodstream, clear the spaces between cells and carry away toxins and foreign particles such as bacteria, cholesterol and viruses. The white cells called lymphocytes that circulate in and out of the lymphatics are an integral part of the body's immune system fighting infection and disease.

The system parallels the blood circulation but with one major difference – it has no central pump like the heart. The movement of lymph relies upon pressure from the normal activity of the surrounding muscles. A sedentary lifestyle can lead to sluggish circulation of lymph.

A healthy lymphatic system can help prevent arteriosclerosis – the thickening and hardening of the arteries. If the lymphatics are blocked, the cholesterol remains in the walls of the arteries, slowing down blood supply to and from the heart.

Deep stress affects the lymphatic system, making us particularly vulnerable to viral infections.

EXERCISE keeps lymph flowing. Muscles are strengthened and their movement pushes the lymph around the body. YOGA is particularly beneficial, reducing stress and relaxing the body. A diet heavy in fats places a burden on the lymphatic system – after a fatty meal, much of the fat ends up in the lymphatics.

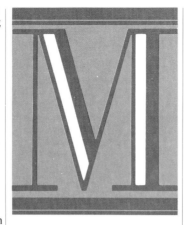

MACROBIOTICS

Macrobiotics is based on the ancient Chinese principle that all life can be viewed as a balance between two energies, Yin and Yang. Yin is associated with cold, rest, responsiveness, passivity, darkness and nourishment. Yang is associated with heat, movement, excitement, upwardness and increase. These aspects are manifest in all areas of life: woman is Yin, man is Yang; night is Yin, day is Yang; most meat is Yang, fruits are Yin.

A macrobiotic diet is a beneficial one – it does not include refined foods and reduces the intake of stimulants, but often includes large amounts of salt and some soya foods. The macrobiotic diet does tend to be low in vitamins B and C, so it is not suitable for young children or babies.

MASKS

There are a variety of masks on the market to suit all types of skins and to perform all sorts of tasks. A mask can deep cleanse, tone, exfoliate, stimulate circulation or moisturise.

Apply a mask when you have at least 30 minutes to relax and lie down. Before applying, cleanse your face, or better still steam it to cleanse and open pores. Follow mask instructions and avoid the eye area.

There are several types of masks…

● Traditional mud setting pack: clay-based and usually dry on the skin. it absorbs excess oil and lifts out dirt from skin's pores. Apply mask to oily areas only. Do not use if you have THREAD VEINS or on dry, sensitive skin.
● Mineral masks: usually contain algae/seaweed to revitalise. Use for sensitive and mature skins.
● Herbal masks: effect depends entirely on the herb used. Azuline, a derivative of camomile, is ideal for sensitive, vascular skin.
Rosemary acts as a stimulant, detoxifying and clearing out congested pores.
● Gels and creams: these have a high water content and are best for dehydrated skins. Can be used several times a week.
● Peel-off masks: applied with a brush or fingertips and left to set on the skin, these masks are finally peeled off taking surface dirt and dead cells with them. They are available for all skin types.

HOME-MADE MASKS

Masks can be made up at home with ingredients from your kitchen cupboard and fridge. They smell good enough to eat! But always make sure home-made face packs use only fresh raw materials and are prepared immediately before use.

How about apples? Excellent for dry skin. Finely grate an apple and add half a teaspoonful of milk and a tablespoon of honey.

Mashed cucumber makes a wonderful cooling and toning mask. Wonderful for summer.

Strawberries pulped with a little milk and cooked mashed potatoes to make a paste leaves your skin smooth and glowing. Leave on face for 30 minutes, then rinse off with lukewarm water.

Brewer's yeast powder isn't so delicious, but it'll give your skin a boost! Dissolve half a teaspoonful of yeast powder in a little water and add a tablespoonful of honey and vegetable oil, and half a teaspoonful of cider vinegar.

If skin is greasy, add a tablespoonful of yoghurt, buttermilk or whipped egg white. For dry skins, add a tablespoon of sour cream and one beaten egg yolk. Mix. Apply a thin coating of oil to the face and apply mask. Leave for 20 minutes.

Fruit pulp masks are refreshing. Use apricot, banana, tomato or strawberry pulp mixed with egg white (two tablespoons of pulp to one egg white), thicken with wheat flour. Leave on face for 20 minutes. Rinse with warm water.

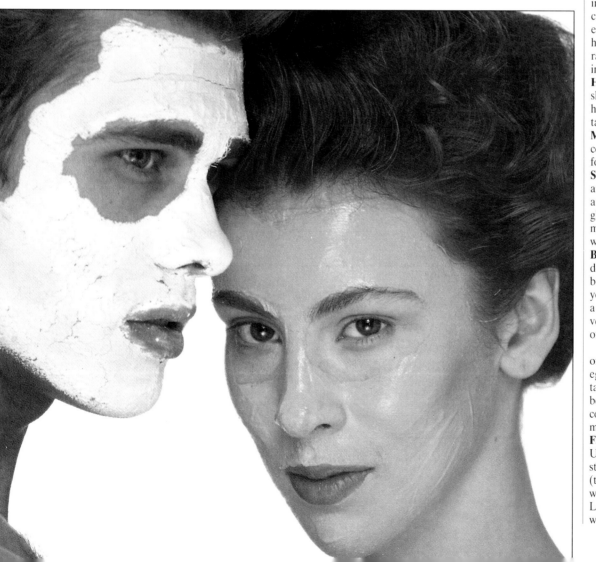

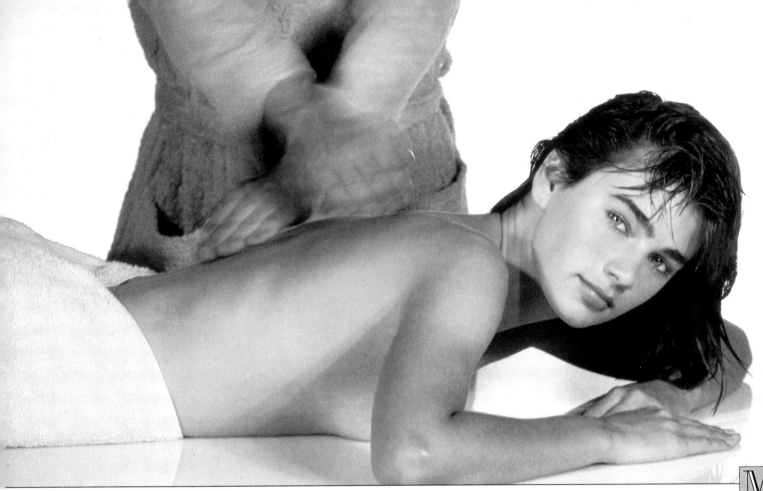

MASSAGE

Touch is a primitive instinct. When a child falls over, mother will 'rub it better'. We instinctively put our arms reassuringly around someone crying or in pain. Rubbing a painful part of the body encourages blood into the area to heal and eases pain. Giving someone a hug communicates sympathy and caring in a way that words cannot. Massage combines both these healing and therapeutic elements of touch. It not only affects a person physically, but induces emotional and mental well-being.

A recent study of premature babies in America showed that massage of the babies by their mothers increased nerve and brain cell development, accelerated weight gain and increased hormonal functioning and cell activity.

Through stroking, pressure and kneading, massage tones muscles and aids the circulation of blood and lymph. (See CIRCULATION and LYMPHATIC SYSTEM.)

The West is generally out of touch with touch, whereas in the East massage is a part of everyday life, and has been for the past five thousand years. But a growing number of

people are at last realising the healing powers of massage and are discerning that it's an ideal way to combat stress.

When visiting a masseur it is advisable not to eat for two to three hours beforehand. Do not drink alcohol the day before. In the treatment room you should find a massage table or couch, clean towels and linen, and a place where you can undress in privacy. Talc, oil or cream will be used to help hands glide over the skin.

There are many different ways of giving a massage from SHIATSU to various intuitive massages linking mind and body. The masseur may massage your entire body, or treatment may be localised.

After a deep massage you may feel stiff and slightly sore the next day, but a warm relaxing bath followed by a brisk cold shower and towelling will help. Benefits are cumulative so it is advisable to have several treatments.

There are many different types of massage, some mechanical. The Vibro-massage/G5 machine massages by vibration. Vacusage involves a series of vacuum cups and helps stimulate lymphatic drainage. Underwater massage involves powerful jets of water directed at specific areas of your body while lying in a special bath. Whirlpools, such as

Jacuzzis, work on the underwater massage principle and are relaxing and toning.

Massage should be a natural part of everyday life and benefit both the giver and receiver. Do not give a massage if you are feeling unwell or tired. Do not massage anyone who is ill without consulting a professionally qualified person. Do not massage bone fractures within six months of an injury.

The massage should be carried out in a warm and quiet room, preferably with soft lighting, either on the floor or on a table covered with foam and a large towel.

These are the basic massage techniques which will help you get back in touch with touch. It's a good idea, though, to have a professional massage yourself before trying it out on someone else. Massage a friend, or get a friend to massage you. It's the ultimate gift.

GLIDING

The commonest of massage strokes. Good for long stretches of muscles. Extend hands, close fingers, relax. Glide along the length of the muscles in the direction of the heart. Do not resist the natural contours of the body. The longer the stroke, the lighter it is; the shorter, the deeper. Remember – shorter strokes are

sedating, faster strokes are stimulating.

Keep the lubricant to hand and if you are using oil, warm it in your cupped palm before applying to the skin. Apply to each area as you work on it. Gliding strokes relax and stretch the muscles in preparation for kneading.

KNEADING

Deeper than gliding. This method is very good for legs, buttocks, back and upper chest. Place heels of hands on the midline of area to be worked. Fingers should be outstretched and relaxed. Push heel and palm of each hand alternately in the direction of the fingers.

FRICTION

Used mainly for the back on knots of tension or areas of stiffness. Always follow with gentle gliding. Using pad of thumb or index finger, slowly apply pressure to the point. Rotate pad slightly or move back and forth for ten-15 seconds before releasing slowly. Repeat not more than three times.

CHOPPING

For calves, upper legs, buttocks. Not for bony areas. The outer edge of the palms and little fingers alternately strike the skin. Fingers, and hands should always be relaxed – almost limp – and shouldn't be raised more than three inches.

CUPPING

Good for the back. Cup hands with fingers and thumbs closed tight enough to hold water. Strike body rhythmically with hollowed palms. Wrists should remain as loose as possible.

Massage a headache away

Throw away the aspirin and find a caring friend. Headaches are invariably caused by tension in the neck and shoulders, so concentrate on knotted muscles in these areas. Finish by massaging the face, especially forehead and temple area. Don't forget the scalp!

Cramp

Don't just concentrate on cramped muscle. If cramp is in the upper arm, for example, massage the whole arm. Use gliding and kneading strokes. End with chopping strokes to stimulate blood supply.
(See ACUPRESSURE, AROMATHERAPY, SHIATSU, STRESS.)

MEDICATION

Medication is used by 'allopathic' medicine (orthodox medicine) to neutralise or oppose a disease. The drugs used do not uproot the causal processes that underlie the disease. Certain diseases – such as those associated with glandular deficiency, like diabetes – are effectively treated by certain drugs. Medication can also suppress diseases of exhaustion and intolerance, such as depression and asthma, until their cause can be dealt with – a good short-term measure. It will also postpone failure of the heart, lungs or kidneys and makes surgery possible.

It is widely known that some drugs can produce side-effects as unpleasant as the symptoms they are treating. Some, such as tranquillisers, have proved addictive, while others, such as antibiotics, can rob the body of certain vitamins.

Used in moderation and under certain circumstances, today's high-tech drugs can make a positive contribution to your health. But they are not a cure-all. Your state of health depends on *you*, and a balanced holistic attitude to your own well-being. Prevention is far better than cure by pill popping!

So start exercising, overhaul your diet, revise your mental and emotional attitudes to life. (See AEROBICS, DIET, EMOTIONS, HOLISTIC.)

MEDITATION

According to ancient traditions of meditation, we all have the capacity to interact with a higher level of being, an inner self that is a source of wisdom and guidance. Our lifestyle today leaves little time for us to contemplate and touch that centre of stillness – we are generally too busy anxiously chasing goals, planning, rushing around, busying ourselves in a world of constant sensory stimulation.

Meditation is the key to this centre of stillness within yourself. It unlocks a permanent sanctuary which can be entered whenever you feel tired, confused, overburdened and stressed. You leave refreshed and with renewed vitality.

Putting time aside each day for meditation helps to quieten the mind, and teaches ways to control, rather than be controlled by, our thoughts and emotions. By learning simple meditation techniques we can enter a state of deep stillness and passive awareness – similar to that between sleep and wakefulness.

Meditation developed as a spiritual practice over 3,000 years ago in the East and the best known method – YOGA – is a means of uniting with Brahman the Absolute. But increasing numbers of people in the West are using meditation without any religious context, as a practical tool for relaxation.

According to research findings, meditation benefits us physically as well as psychologically. It quietens the sympathetic nervous system, slows the breathing rate and heartbeat, and lowers blood pressure and metabolism. Various ailments, especially those which are stress-related – such as phobias, nervous tension, disturbed sleep, high blood pressure and drug and alcohol dependencies – benefit from meditation.

There are many types of meditation. Yoga uses the breath – prana – to exert control over pain, emotions and physical health, and the body is gently stretched to hold certain positions. There is a sense of surrender to the physical body for release of emotional, mental and bodily tensions.

Zazen and Vispassana, known as insight meditation, demand complete immobility, concentrating attention on the rise and fall of the abdomen as you breathe. This type of meditation can bring up repressed feelings which have been stifling creative and emotional fulfilment.

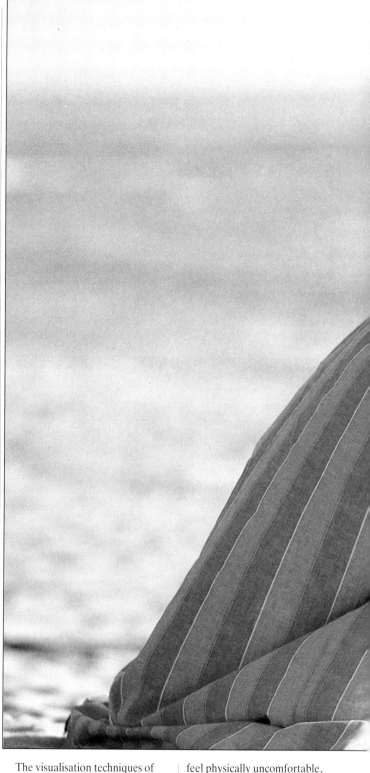

The visualisation techniques of Tibetan Buddhism focus the mind on a particular image, while other meditative practices focus on the repetition chanting of a particular word or phrase.

The most simple meditation techniques can easily become part of an everyday routine. Set aside two periods of ten to 20 minutes for meditation each day, preferably in the morning and in the evening. When you start to meditate you may feel physically uncomfortable, nauseous, anxious or agitated – if so, stop meditating, open your eyes and relax again. When you feel better, resume meditation.

Sometimes, thoughts and images from the unconscious mind reveal themselves. They may be parts of ourselves which we find frightening, embarrassing or uncomfortable, but they soon fade once they are recognised. Don't be discouraged if you find your mind wandering during

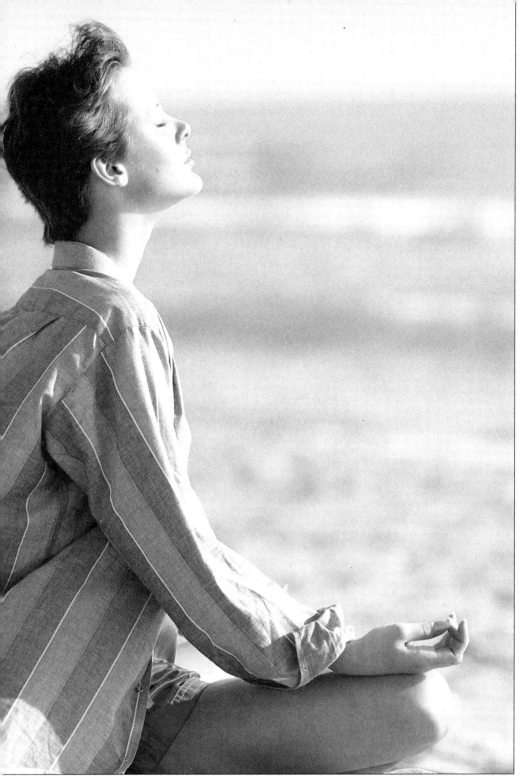

After meditation

Do not get up suddenly. Stretch gently and move around slowly. You should feel refreshed and relaxed, but persevere if you don't notice results immediately – after a week you are almost sure to feel the benefits.

MELANOMA

Melanoma is the most serious form of skin cancer. It is mainly caused by intermittent exposure of unprepared skin to ultraviolet sunlight, especially in fair-skinned people. Early detection is crucial. Approximately half of all melanomas occur on previously non-malignant black or brown moles or birthmarks.

Always wear a high-factor sunscreen, whatever your skin type, throughout the year. (See TANNING, SUN.)

Consult your doctor immediately if you notice any of the following changes in moles or birthmarks…

● Increase in size
● Itching
● Inflammation
● Irregular outline
● Change in colour
● Crusting or bleeding
● Moles or marks measuring more than one centimetre across
● Sudden coarse hair growth in the mole

MENOPAUSE

This is the time in a woman's life when menstruation ceases. Production of the hormones oestrogen and progesterone wind down, causing menstrual flow to decrease accordingly. This shift to a new hormonal balance can often lead to erratic periods.

Every woman experiences menopause differently. For some, menstruation ends abruptly at any time from the early 40s onwards – although menopause can occur earlier. But for most it is a gradual slowing down of ovarian function, spanning up to ten years. Many women seem hardly aware that it is happening, while others suffer a variety of problems which they associate with the menopause.

Menopause, like menstrual onset, is fraught with rumour and misunderstanding. It is often seen as a negative development in a woman's life, when, in fact, menopause is a positive and natural transitional period into another phase in female maturity. It is the beginning of an

---

meditation; this is normal and will eventually stop after practice.

Getting ready
● Take the phone off the hook, find a quiet, comfortable spot to relax.
● Get into a position that allows you to sit comfortably erect without strain.
● Close your eyes, take several slow deep breaths. Lay your hands on your abdomen and breathe in deeply, filling your stomach first. Sigh as you breathe out releasing tension in the

feet first, then with the next exhalation, the ankles, then calves and so on.
● Contact each part of your body with your mind and release it completely before moving on to the next stage.

Meditating
Focused breathing method
Focus on the rise and fall of your abdomen or on the air flowing through your nostrils. If you find it

difficult to concentrate on your breathing, silently count each breath from one to ten.

Mantra meditation
Silently repeat a word or phrase that you like. 'Peace' is a popular mantra.

Concentrative meditation
Focus without blinking on a static, small object about a metre away, then close your eyes and try to visualise it. When the after-image fades away, start again.

exciting and challenging stage of life.

Research shows that the only symptoms directly caused by a reduction in female hormone production are hot flushes, osteoporosis and vaginal dryness but menopause is associated with hot flushes, vaginal dryness, weight gain, wrinkles, thinning hair, unwanted facial hair, osteoporosis, depression, anxiety and even madness. In cultures where menopause is embraced as a welcome passage in life and post-menopausal women are respected for their wisdom and experience, women rarely complain of unpleasant symptoms.

A sense of feeling unwanted and redundant can trigger the symptoms generally associated with menopause, especially depression. Studies have shown that women who have devoted themselves to childbearing and housework are more likely to be adversely affected by menopause than those with personal sources of satisfaction outside the home.

HORMONE REPLACEMENT THERAPY often is the most successful way to deal with severe problems in menopause. Women on HRT should be constantly supervised and monitored by their doctor. However there are other ways of managing menopausal side effects.

HOT FLUSHES

These can be very distressing and embarrassing. They last from 15 seconds to a minute – face and neck suddenly turn a bright red, and the flushes are often accompanied by sweating and a tingling sensation in the fingers and toes.

Try to avoid meat and poultry in your diet as these may contain residues of steroid growth promoters which, along with stimulants such as coffee, alcohol and smoking, will aggravate the condition.

If flushes continue, take between 200-400 IU of vitamin E with 1000 mg of vitamin C daily.

OSTEOPOROSIS

A quarter of all menopausal women suffer from osteoporosis, which is believed to be preventable by taking plenty of exercise and increasing calcium in your diet (cheese, milk, tofu, turnip greens, soya beans, almonds, brazil nuts, yoghurt, shrimps, tinned salmon, tinned sardines). (See OSTEOPOROSIS.)

SEX

It is not true that sex becomes more difficult during menopause. Most women who enjoy an active and fulfilling sex life before menopause

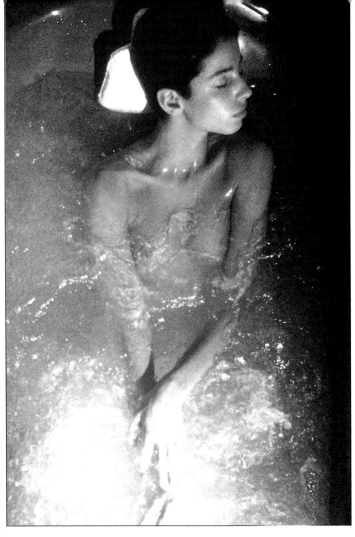

continue to do so during and afterwards. In fact, many women report an increase in libido – probably due to a potent combination of experience, self-knowledge and confidence that comes with middle age. Any vaginal dryness can be countered by using lubricants such as KY jelly.

It is still possible to get pregnant during menopause. You can still ovulate, even though you have missed several periods. A test for hormones in the blood will tell you whether you should continue with contraception.

For menopausal health take supplements of Evening Primrose Oil, calcium and vitamin B complex. Fennel tea contains plant oestrogens.

Menopause is a gateway to a new freedom, and offers an ideal opportunity for a reappraisal of your lifestyle. What would you like to change? Is there anything in your relationships you would like to change? Is there anything you've always wanted to do, but never dared to, or didn't have the time for? It is an ideal time for taking up new interests, for travelling, for making new friends. The more fulfilled you are, the more likely menopause will be a

phase of life to be welcomed rather than feared.

MENSTRUATION

Baby girls are born with up to half a million eggs (ova). From puberty until menopause an ovum is released each month from one or other ovary and finds its way into the adjacent Fallopian tube. But before release the ovum ripens in a sort of shell called the Graafian follicle. The ovum is released by the follicle which remains behind and grows into a small endocrine gland, the corpus luteum. This produces the hormone progesterone which stimulates the lining of the uterus to thicken and prepare itself to receive a fertilised egg (embryo).

If the ovum is not fertilised, production of progesterone by the corpus luteum ceases and the uterus sheds its lining. The raw surface bleeds a little   approximately two ounces (600cc) of blood is lost during the menstrual period.

The menstrual cycle is a unique opportunity for every woman to tune

All of the following change during menstruation

Blood sugar levels
Rectal and vaginal temperatures
Metabolism
Water retention
Body weight
Arterial oxygen pressure
Blood acidity
Heartbeat
Blood leucocyte counts
Platelet counts
Vitamins A C and E requirements
Bile pigments
Urine volume
Skin colour and permeability
Cervix
Smelling ability
Pain threshold
Psychic activities
Dreams
Thyroid and adrenaline function

in to how her body works, to get in touch with her body's rhythms. The most common cycle runs 28 days – parallel to the cycle of the moon – but it can vary from 24 to 32 days.

You can learn a lot about yourself by keeping a careful record for three months: note the first day of every period on a calendar and chart your moods and feelings each day. Count the days between periods. If your first sighting of blood was December 1 and your next period begins on December 30th, your cycle is 29 days. Also note your time of ovulation – beforehand your temperature will drop sharply followed by a sharp rise the next day. Cervical mucus becomes transparent and elastic like raw egg white before ovulation.

Knowing when you ovulate is useful if you want to use the natural birth control method. (See CONTRACEPTION.) And for many women it's a time when they feel a surge of creativity, are introspective and energy levels rise or fall.

Getting in touch with your cycle means you can enjoy the different stages and plan ahead positively.

If you feel specially creative during ovulation, set aside time for your favourite creative pursuit. Listen, watch and chart your body. Your dream patterns may change and dreams can be more intense just before and during menstruation; both intuitive and psychic powers may be heightened.

Your menstrual cycle can be used positively and is a way of getting in touch with yourself and inhabiting the kingdom of your body.

Illness, emotional upset,

unexpected irregular sex, travel, fatigue and stress can all affect the menstrual cycle.

MENSTRUAL TIPS

⬤ The ESSENTIAL OILS marjoram, lavender and camomile used either in massage or in baths help ease menstrual cramps and pelvic congestion. so can orgasms. (See AROMATHERAPY, BATHING.)

⬤ Use shiatsu to counteract period pains – with pads of both thumbs press hard for 15 seconds on sole of the foot, a third of the distance from the tip of the middle toe to the heel, between the second and third toe joints.

⬤ Avoid alcohol while bleeding, especially red wine.

⬤ Don't feel guilty because you feel tired. Indulge your need to sleep whenever you can.

⬤ Cycling is the best menstrual exercise – it relieves congestion, that dull ache and cramps. Combine your favourite exercise with plenty of stretching.

⬤ Step up your intake of iron while bleeding – eat plenty of green leafy vegetables, beetroot, cherries, blackcurrants, seeds, offal, free-range eggs, watercress and dried apricots.

⬤ Drink lots of water.

⬤ You may need extra support during this time – share that need with your family and loved ones.

⬤ More than any other bodily function menstruation is associated with myths and taboos rooted in centuries of ignorance.

Women need to have a positive attitude to their cycle to counter the negative attitude of society generally. It will add to your confidence and pride in being a woman.

MINERALS

Minerals are metallic and non-metallic elements found in soil and the sea. We obtain them from the plants and animals we eat.

Macro-minerals are required by the body in quantities of several hundred milligrams per day and are involved in structural functions such as bones and cells as well as the body's metabolism. They include calcium, phosphorus, magnesium, sodium, potassium and chlorine.

The trace elements include iron, zinc, copper, manganese, iodine, selenium, molybdenum and cobalt. They are crucial contributors to the body's metabolism, and are required in smaller daily quantities.

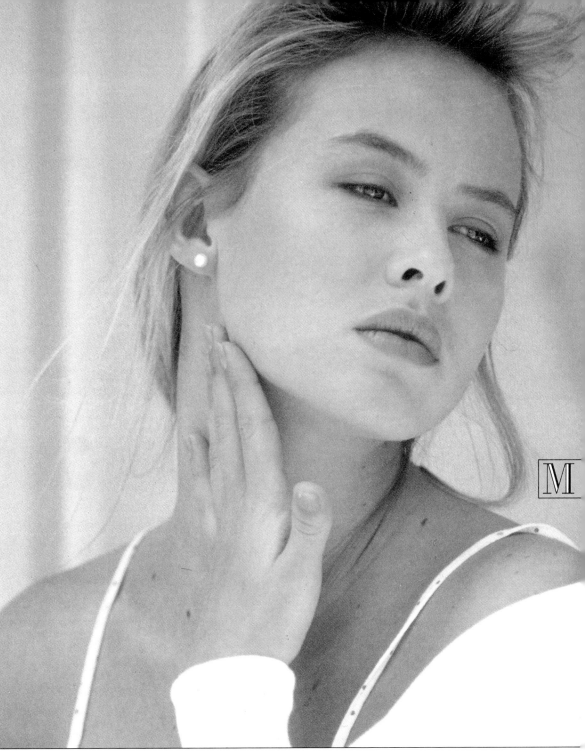

M

WHERE TO FIND MACRO-MINERALS

Calcium: almonds, brazil nuts, caviar, kelp, milk and milk products, tinned salmon, tinned sardines, shrimps, soya beans, tofu, turnip and yoghurt

Chlorine: kelp, olives, sea salt, table salt, salt substitutes.

Magnesium: almonds, bluefish, carp, cod, flounder, halibut, herring, leafy green vegetables, mackerel, molasses, nuts, shrimps, snails, soya beans, sunflower seeds, wheatgerm, corn, dark green vegetables

Phosphorus: almonds, dried beans, calves' liver, cheese, eggs, fish, milk and milk products, peanuts, peas, poultry, pumpkin seeds, red meat, sardines, scallops, soya beans, sunflower seeds, tuna, whole grain products

Potassium chloride: avocados, bananas, citrus fruits, lentils, milk, nuts, parsnips, peaches, potatoes, raisins, sardines, spinach, watercress, whole grains

MOISTURISING

Your body is constantly losing moisture through the skin as water in the cells on the skin's surface evaporates into the atmosphere. Lack of skin care and harsh cosmetics, combined with low humidity in the immediate environment, can wreak havoc on skin leaving it dry, dull and rough.

Moisturisers can help by protecting the skin from dirt and polluting elements and, most important of all,

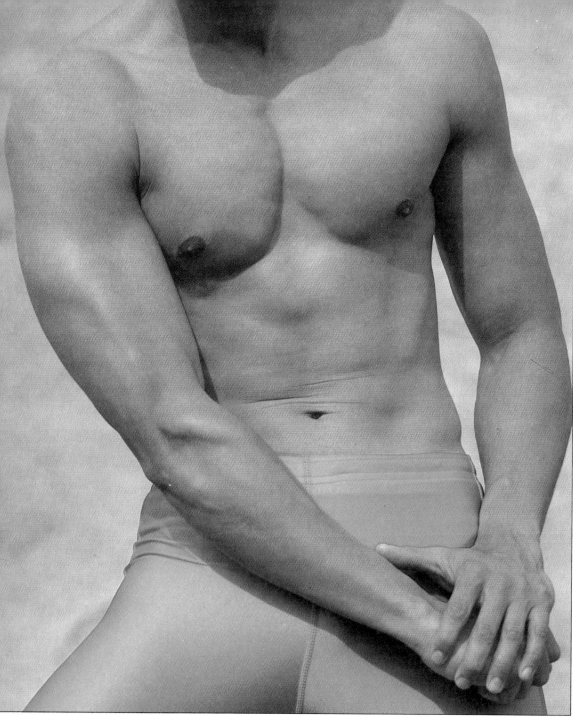

24 hours, which is why regular exercise – especially aerobic activity – is essential for keeping muscles toned and strong.

Your internal organs and skeleton are held in place by your muscles. If muscles are too tense or flaccid, they can distort the shape of your body; weak abdomen muscles allow the stomach and intestines to fall forward, tense muscles in the back and neck pull the spine forward.

Stretching exercises stimulate the flow of blood to and from muscles, essential for cleansing and supplying nutrients. Fifteen minutes of stretching each day gives a lovely sense of release from tension and adds a spring to your step – the whole body feels renewed. The best times for stretching are in the morning and evening (but not immediately before bedtime). Don't rush – take your time. Hold each stretch for 30 seconds so that tension in muscles can be fully released. Breathe deeply throughout each stretch. Here goes.

Waist and spine stretch
Stand and centre your pelvis. Rest hands on shoulders, lengthen your spine and rotate your upper body to the right, keeping the lower half straight.

Hold position for 30 seconds and repeat to left.

Lunge
Stand with the legs apart and the soles of both feet firmly on the floor. Keeping the right leg straight bend the left knee and lunge downwards until you feel a stretch on the inside of the right thigh.

You may include an upper body stretch by raising right arm (as pictured right).

Repeat twice on each side.

by adding moisture to the skin.

Choose a light moisturiser or lotion rather than a heavy cream.

If you have dry skin, use a moisturiser with a vegetable base such as sesame, avocado or olive oil – not mineral oil.

If you have oily skin use a water-based moisturiser.

Men's skin is 24 per cent thicker than women's, is more resilient and produces more sebum (oil) so it needs a lighter moisturiser, preferably a water-in-oil product that feels cool and light. There are a number of moisturisers available specially for men.

Before applying moisturiser,
cleanse skin thoroughly, then use a toning lotion with cold water to close pores. Apply moisturiser when skin is still damp. Use a small amount, massaging in with upward strokes on chin, cheek and forehead and in circular motions into the bridge of the nose. Blot off excess.

You'll need extra moisturiser during the winter, as humidity is lower. Counter the drying effects of central heating with a humidifier or leave a bowl of water in each room to raise the moisture level.

Change your moisturiser in the summer for one that contains PABA (para-amino benzoic acid), which is a natural sunscreen.

MUSCLES

Muscles are the power units of our body that make direct use of energy. They make up over a third of our body weight, and 1,200 of them are directly under our control, while others are involuntary and never stop working – such as the heart and those that keep the digestive tract active.

Muscles are actually bundles of long connecting fibres that exert force by contracting. Muscle tissue is like an engine kept permanently ticking over – even at rest it is in a state of alert. However, it deteriorates quickly if left inactive for longer than

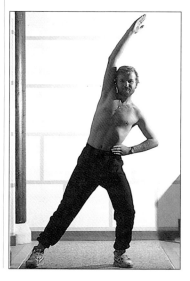

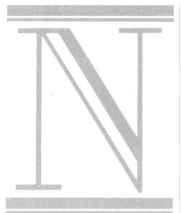

NATUROPATHY

The philosophy of naturopathy is based on three principles:
● The body possesses the power to heal itself through its own internal vitality.
● Disease is the body's way of removing obstruction to normal function.
● Disease affects the whole organism, not simply the isolated organ or system. Naturopathy treats the whole person and not just the symptoms. (See HOLISTIC.)

Naturopathy has evolved by observation and application over thousands of years, but the word naturopathy has only been used since the beginning of this century. Its aim is to promote health, rather than confront disease, and to educate people to adopt a healthy lifestyle.

Some basic naturopathic principles can be observed in the instinctive behaviour of animals – they seek warmth when chilled, try to cool inflamed parts.

In Ancient Greece Hippocrates, the father of medicine, recognised the power of nature's own healing abilities. For instance, he believed fever to be a manifestation of healing at work.

Naturopathy has long recognised that DIET plays an essential part in maintaining health – 'let food be your medicine and let medicine be your food'.

Modern research confirms this: lack of certain nutrients such as proteins and an excess of inappropriate foods such as sugar have been shown to create biochemical and metabolic changes which can result in a wide variety of physical, emotional and mental symptoms

On your first visit a naturopath will build up your unique health profile by noting your flavour cravings and response to crises, change and

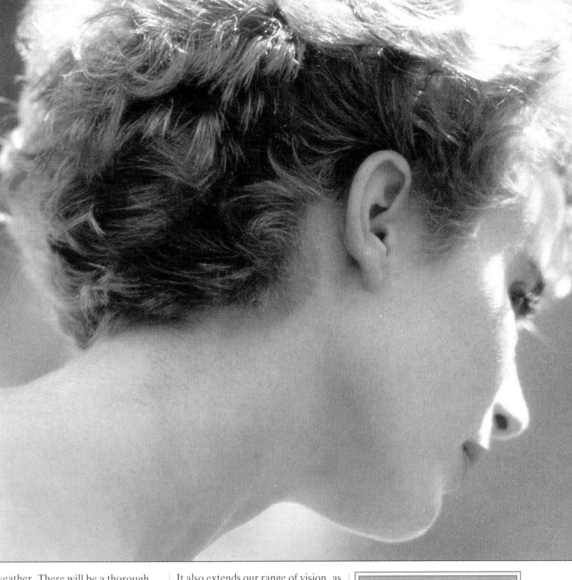

weather. There will be a thorough physical examination and other skills may be used such as IRIDOLOGY (the study of the iris) to build up a thorough picture of your health. A small amount of your hair may be sent away for mineral content analysis. Changes in diet will be recommended, and supplements prescribed. You may also be advised to carry out some HYDROTHERAPY practices at home involving BATHING, COMPRESSES, and sprays, and introduced to relaxation techniques. Naturopathy recognises the importance of mental and emotional well-being, so psychological counselling is often a vital component of naturopathic treatment.

NECK

The neck not only supports the weight of our head, but houses the larynx (voice box) and seven vertebrae with a number of complex muscles attached in front and behind.

It also extends our range of vision, as any tennis spectator will know.

As a 'bridge' between the brain and the body, the neck often harbours tension. Clenched muscles at the root of the neck around the shoulders and in the neck itself can inhibit mobility and restrict blood flow to the head, causing headaches and stiffness.

Any neck pain that travels down one arm should be reported to a doctor immediately.

The following exercises won't eliminate neck tension, but will control it . . .
● Look straight ahead, turn your head to the right until your nose lines up with your right shoulder; repeat to the left. Repeat several times a day, or whenever you feel your neck tensing.
● Circle the points of both shoulders forward, up, back and down – both together, then separately.

Any gentle massage of the neck and shoulders can help with tension headaches, or place cold COMPRESSES to the forehead and back of the neck, or hot and cold compresses on the

NECK CARE

DO concentrate on your posture – it's vital. Check in the mirror that head is directly above shoulders, not in front
DO support your neck with a suitably comfortable pillow in bed
DO gentle neck exercises regularly to avoid stiffness
DON'T scrunch your neck over steering wheel while driving
DON'T slouch while sitting
DON'T lie on a high pillow
DON'T sleep on your stomach

back of the neck and shoulders.

The skin on the neck needs as much care and attention as the skin on your face. When using a moisturiser make sure you massage well into your neck, and when treating yourself to a face pack, include the back and front of the neck.

When taking a bath containing an essential oil, immerse your neck in the water if you can.

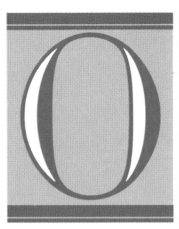

OSTEOPATHY

Osteopathy is concerned with the structural and mechanical problems of the body. It deals with the body's entire framework including bones, joints, muscles, ligaments and other supportive soft tissues. Its aim is to restore ease of movement and functioning by manual pressure.

Modern osteopathic philosophy and practice are founded on the concept that our normal state of being is healthy. Treatment and diagnosis are based on three fundamental principles:
● The body's natural tendency is to heal itself.
● An intimate relationship between structure and function – ie between the movement of a joint and the workings of the smallest cell.
● The body has a better chance of functioning at all levels if it is structurally and mechanically sound.

The spinal cord can be seen as an extension of the brain, linking to all the major organs via the nervous system. Osteopathic practice believes that any interference with the spinal cord – for example, through bad posture, pull of gravity and stress – can affect the normal functions of tissues to which the nerves are connected, including major organs such as the heart, kidneys and liver.

So, as well as successfully treating structural disorders such as arthritis, joint pains and sports injuries, osteopathy may also be used to treat asthma, respiratory problems, headaches, digestive disorders, period pains and poor circulation. Correct medical advice, and treatment where necessary, should also be sought for such disorders.

A typical osteopathic treatment of lower back pain may consist of small rhythmical movements to the lower spine to stretch the contracted tissues. Gentle pressure is then applied to painful muscles to encourage relaxation. If a joint has lost some of its mobility, the osteopath will 'gap' the joint surfaces – the joint is quickly and painlessly taken through its range of movement. Don't be alarmed if you hear a loud click – that's normal.

OSTEOPOROSIS

Thinning of the texture of the bone – known as osteoporosis – is most common in menopausal and post-menopausal white women and is the cause of frequent fractures of bones,
deformed spinal column (known as dowager's hump) and loss of height. Several factors play a part in the gradual onset of osteoporosis . . .

Bones help maintain the levels of the calcium in the blood. When the level drops below a certain point, calcium stored in the bones is used up (resorption). When the calcium level in the blood rises, it is either excreted or reabsorbed into the bones. This process of absorption and resorption stays roughly in balance until early middle age when resorption increases.

The decline in the production of the female hormone oestrogen during menopause affects the body's ability to absorb calcium, which is why the calcium content in the bones of women over 35 decreases by one per cent per year.

Bone mass thins most dramatically during the three to seven years after menopause and, if combined with inactivity, poor nutrition, or a build up of lead and aluminium in the bones, can cause bones to break easily and spontaneously, particularly in old age.

Osteoporosis is not an inevitable part of old age. It can be prevented, and the earlier you start taking precautions the better. Studies both here and in the USA show that it is never too late to improve the quality of your skeleton. Bone is highly responsive to the right stimuli and quickly increases density when you combine the following . . .
● Supplement your diet with calcium. Milk, as everyone knows, is a good source of calcium along with all other dairy products. But to get the daily
requirement of 1500mg of calcium you would need to drink at least three glasses a day. This could leave you with a weight problem, so you may prefer to supplement your diet with calcium in tablet form. Or, better still, eat plenty of calcium-packed alternatives, such as sardines, shellfish, oats, pulses and nuts.
● Make sure enough vitamin D is included in your diet. It helps the body absorb calcium, getting it into the digestive tract and into the bones. Sunlight is an excellent source of vitamin D, but we don't get enough of it in northern Europe.

Concentrate on including natural sources of vitamin D in your diet – cod-liver oil is an excellent source and can be taken daily in capsule form. Herring, mackerel, salmon and herring all contain vitamin D. Magnesium too, found in beans, nuts, cereals and seafoodaids calcium absorption.
● Exercise regularly. Concentrate on any of the weight-bearing exercises, such as walking. No matter how old you are, exercise increases mineralisation of bone. Like muscle, bone grows stronger as greater demands are placed upon it. Post-menopausal women can continue to build their bones instead of losing them if they exercise regularly. (See EXERCISE, AEROBICS, FITNESS.)
● Oestrogen supplements may also reduce loss in bone density. (See HORMONE REPLACEMENT THERAPY.) Smokers get osteoporosis sooner; smoking hastens menopause and its drop in oestrogen levels, advancing the onset of osteoporosis by as much as five years.

OVERWEIGHT

In our society slimness is a symbol of all that is meant to be desirable – success, self-control, health, beauty and social acceptability.

It is possible to be fat and still have all these things, except good health. Extra weight increases the risk of serious disorders such as high blood pressure, diabetes and heart disease.

Overweight people live shorter lives, are ill more often, and, in extreme cases, are subject to the added stress of being ridiculed because of their obesity.

Extra body fat is created mainly because more food energy is being consumed than is being expended. The body stores the excess food energy as fat. Energy-saving elements of modern life, such as cars, lifts, escalators, and sedentary work all

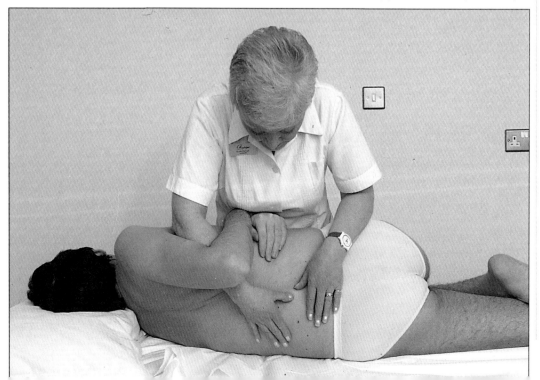

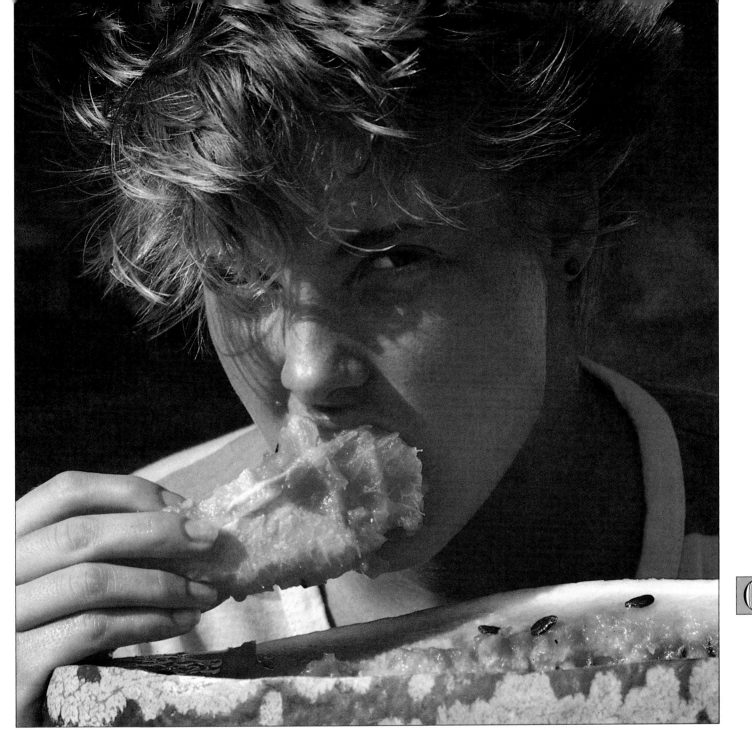

conspire to keep calories piling up.

The solution seems simple: consume fewer calories so you *eat less;* burn more calories – so you *exercise more.*

Unfortunately, as most overweight or recently slimmed people will admit, losing weight is not easy. Crash fad diets are rarely the best way of doing it, as they tend to ignore the underlying psychological reasons for overeating and are usually ineffective unless combined with a regular exercise programme.

The first step on the road to losing weight is to understand the underlying reasons why you overeat.

You may be trying to hide your sexual attractiveness, you may be bored or lonely, insecure, your self-esteem may be extremely low. Counselling and psychotherapy can help unearth the psychological factors.

Once you've decided to cut calories and launch into a regular exercise programme, remember to . . .
● Keep busy. Plan a busy social life, and take up new interests. Boredom will have you heading for the fridge.
● Replace lunch and dinner dates with interesting outings.
● Drink plenty of water – up to eight glasses a day. Water fills you up and doesn't contain one single calorie.

● Only eat when you are hungry.
● Take it easy. As you lose weight, you may feel more tired. Don't think that because you are losing weight you can do more. You can't – not yet!
● Resist cravings. Your mind is your ally and will help you if you let it. Through meditation, deep relaxation or an hypnotic state you can beat those unhealthy desires for, say, chocolate. While meditating or in a relaxed state, visualise the masticated chocolate glued into disgusting fat deposits on your stomach. Then imagine yourself trim and fit – as you would like to be. Imagine what you would wear and how you would feel

and move. (See MEDITATION. RELAXATION. CRAVINGS.)

Put meals on smaller plates to give the illusion that you're eating more

Use measured quantities of food

Always sit at the table and don't read or watch television while eating – you'll be distracted and eat more than you want

Put down knife and fork between each bite

Chew each morsel 20 times

Don't put more food in your mouth until what you are eating is swallowed

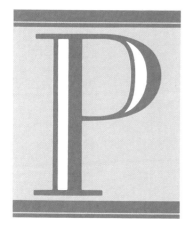

PAIN

Pain is the body's warning system and its most dramatic way of telling you that something is wrong. Endorphins, the body's natural painkillers, are released by pain, stress and exercise. If you are in pain, relaxation techniques and correct breathing can help.

Deep relaxation techniques are increasingly being used rather than drugs, to overcome pain, and the effects can be long lasting without unwanted side effects.

LAUGHTER, ACUPUNCTURE and REFLEXOLOGY all help ease pain – they are believed to release endorphins too. HYPNOTHERAPY can help you to live with constant pain by changing your attitude to it, and can also increase endorphin levels.

Trypotophan, an essential amino acid, alters pain receptors in the brain and can raise pain tolerance. It can be found in soya beans, wheatgerm and sesame seeds, and works best when taken in conjunction with a low protein diet. (See AMINO ACIDS.)

Studies of acutely ill medical patients in the USA link low magnesium levels with low pain tolerance.

Foods rich in magnesium include wholemeal bread, shrimps, bananas, black treacle, nuts, peas and soya beans. (See MINERALS.)

PETS

Keeping pets can make a positive contribution to our physical and emotional health. Studies show that the heartbeat drops and blood pressure lowers while stroking an animal, and the therapeutic value of touch is already well established. For many people living alone, or with communication

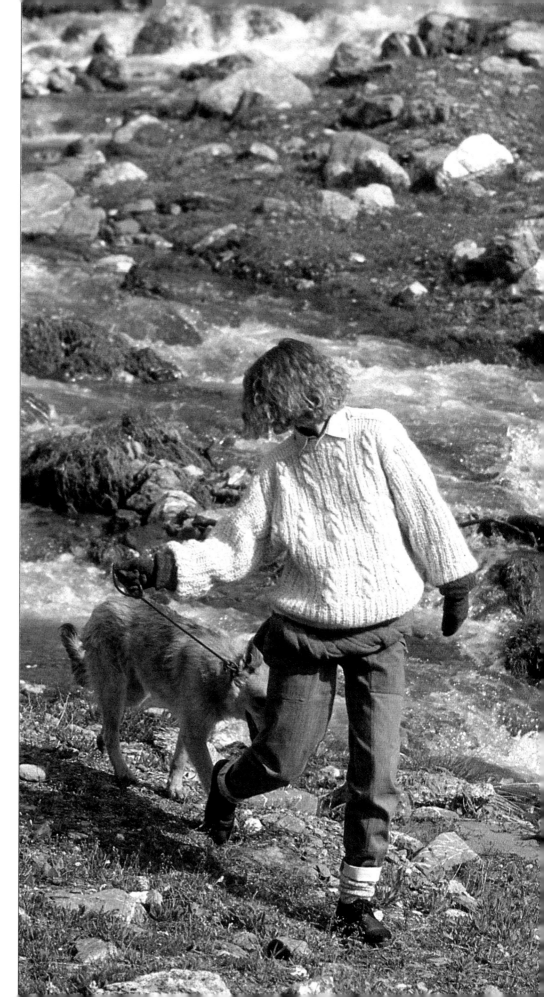

difficulties, pets can be the only source of loving touch and often the only company during the day.

A brisk half-hour walk with the dog twice a day is an excellent form of aerobic exercise, and will keep your heart and lungs healthy as well as your dog's.

Careful attention to your pet's hygiene, and simple rules such as never allowing pets in the bedroom, and keeping them out of the kitchen when food is being prepared can minimise infections caught by humans from animals.

Never let your dog foul in public places – dog faeces are a source of several unpleasant diseases.

POLLUTION

Our environment is polluted by a variety of toxic substances which affect our health. We breathe polluted air, eat food which has been processed with chemicals, and drink polluted water which depletes the body's supply of vitamins – especially A, C, E and the B VITAMINS. Poisonous heavy metals such as lead, aluminium and mercury can upset the mineral balance.

Anti-pollution nutrients can help protect the body from the ravages of various toxins, so include them in your DIET and as SUPPLEMENTS if necessary.

Research shows that natural FIBRE helps flush out pollutants such as lead and cadmium and helps remove radioactive strontium from the body.

Vitamin A helps prevent damage caused by nitrogen oxide present in car exhaust and cigarette smoke. The vitamin regenerates lung tissue damaged by nitrogen oxide. Anyone constantly exposed to urban pollution and who is a regular commuter should take note. Eat plenty of apricots, broccoli, carrots, liver, spinach, sweet potatoes, water melon, mustard greens.

Vitamin E is another anti-oxidant vitamin and helps counteract the effects of nitrogen dioxide, and X-ray radiation. It also protects stores of vitamin A in lung tissue. Sources of vitamin E include margarine, almonds, corn oil, wheatgerm, wholewheat, walnuts, sunflower seeds.

Vitamin C (ascorbic acid) helps detoxify the body of heavy metals, and harmful nitrates (used in chemical fertilisers). Found in most fruits, especially blackcurrants and oranges as well as green peppers, cabbage, brussels sprouts and watercress.

POSITIVE THINKING

Our attitudes dramatically affect the quality of our lives, including our health and our relationships. The way we respond to people and situations determines how pleasant our lives are now and will become in the future.

When we learn to adopt a positive mental attitudes and strong self-esteem we not only find an immense personal benefit, but we can give so much more to those around us and those we love.

Our attitudes have developed from the cradle to the present day – we have been 'programmed' by our experiences. We can 're-programme'. It takes just three steps, *want*, *belief* and *effort*. We have the ability to control what we do, and also what we think and what we feel.

Developing positive mental attitudes can fuel our energy and enthusiasm, charge our imagination and creativity and provide a strong foundation from which to build a healthy, happy, fulfilled life.

THE FIRST STEPS

● It's true! There's no such word as 'can't'. Instead be honest and say, 'I don't want to', or 'I don't know how to yet, but I could learn'.

Say to yourself, 'I can!'

● Beware of the negatives. Don't encourage born moaners. They don't want solutions to their problems, they would rather regularly feed on your sympathy.

Seek the company of positive, enthusiastic people; their attitude is infectious and makes us feel good.

● Fear of failure stops us trying new things. If you try something and make a mess of it, no one is going to throw you in the lion's den! Just pick yourself up and have another go until you learn the skills and gain confidence. Don't give up halfway through a task or problem.

● Don't be an 'if only' person. The basic reasons we do things is either because it gives us pleasure or to avoid having a guilty conscience, or because we do not have the courage to carry out what we would really like to do.

You always have a choice. Blaming someone else may give some short-term comfort, but it keeps us locked into negative situations and emotions.

● Ban cynicism. It may be fashionable in some circles, but it is very negative and destructive to everyone it comes in contact with.

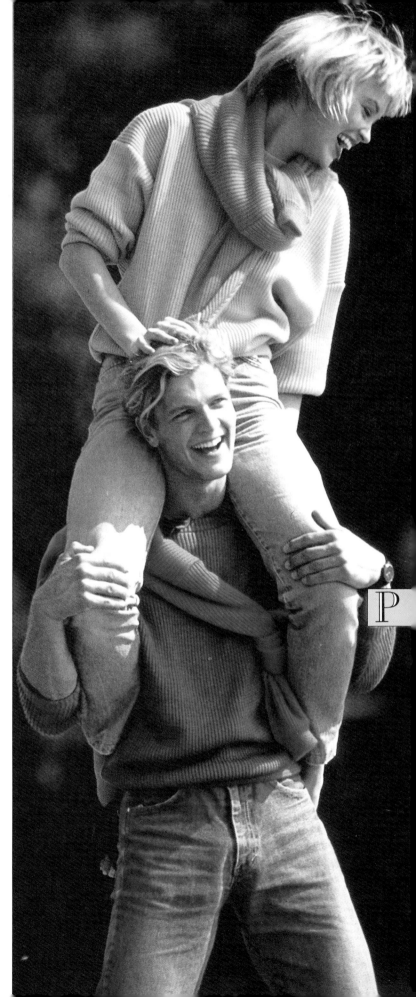

P

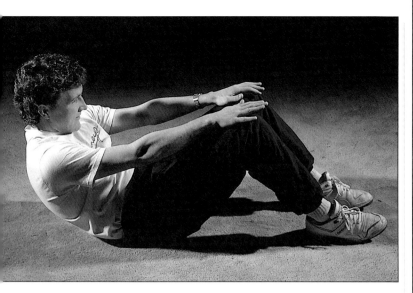

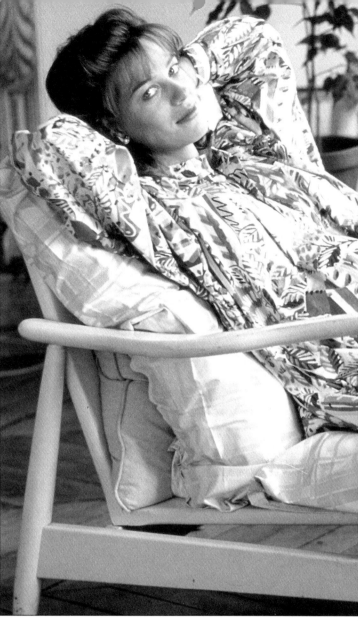

POT BELLY

If, when you look down, you can only see the tips of your toes, or nothing at all except a wobbling mound, you've got a pot belly. In some cultures it's a sign of success and great wealth. In reality it's an indication that your lifestyle needs a major overhaul.

All that extra up-front weight is an added strain on your heart, digestive system, back and knees. Want to get rid of it? Of course you do! Here's what you need to do. . .

● Stop drinking beer as often as you do. Drink only juices or mineral water.

● Start to exercise – very gently at first. Walking is ideal to begin with and swimming is the most comfortable – the water supports your big tummy while you exercise the rest of your body. Remember that for any exercise to be effective it must be taken regularly. A dip in the pool once a month won't help.

● Try the following exercises. The first one you can do several times a day in the car, in your work place or at home.

Sit or stand erect. Pull in stomach as hard as you can with abdominal muscles. Your stomach ought to feel as though it is pressing against your backbone. Count to six slowly and then release and relax.

Repeat 15 times. You should be able to talk and breathe normally while doing this.

Alternatively, try this tummy toner every day. Lie on the floor, knees slightly bent, feet hip-width apart. Roll shoulders up away from floor until you can reach your knees with your fingertips (see above). Repeat ten times, building up to 20.

With the same movement, reach right through between your knees. Repeat six times and when that gets easy, add on 20 elbow-to-opposite-knee touches.

● Take expert advice on your diet. Your doctor is the best person to consult. Don't follow crash diets which promise you'll lose stones in a week. They can be dangerous and once off the diet, you'll very quickly go back to your old weight.

● Avoid late-night meals and don't go to bed on a full stomach. Your body won't be able to burn off calories while you're sleeping.

(See AEROBICS, DIET, EXERCISE, FITNESS, OVERWEIGHT, SLIMMING.)

PREGNANCY

A wanted baby brings the greatest joy, celebration and love. And as parents proudly hold their new son or daughter, they know better than anyone what an exciting and often fearful journey the pregnancy has been. The birth of a healthy baby depends very much on the nine months preceding it. While cradled in the womb, the foetus is extremely sensitive to both the physical and emotional state of the mother (and of the father, to a lesser extent).

If you are planning a baby, your chances of conception will increase if you have a healthy and balanced lifestyle. A nutritious diet, a fit body and a sense of emotional and spiritual well-being are all essential precursors to a perfect, healthy new life and a happy pregnancy.

Avoid drugs of any kind during pregnancy: this includes caffeine, alcohol and cigarettes. Many of the complaints of early pregnancy have been effectively treated by natural methods without recourse to drugs.

● Relax in a bath to which has been added two drops each of lavender, lemon balm or camomile essential oils (or six drops of one) to help constipation. And drink lemon juice in a cup of warm water half an hour before breakfast. Constipation is caused mainly by the increase in the hormone progesterone which relaxes the intestinal muscles, exacerbating varicose veins and piles.

● Some women find feelings of nausea can be eased with fennel tea.

● Morning sickness is believed by some to be nature's message to the mother to rest and prepare for a healthy pregnancy. Whatever the cause, it's very unpleasant. Try any of the following infusions to ease the problem – lemon balm, hops, lavender flowers and camomile flowers. The latter can help contractions and may be drunk before and during labour.

DIET

● Food for pregnancy needs to provide a balance of vitamins, minerals, proteins, carbohydrates and fats, while augmenting those nutrients on which the foetus makes a special demand – particularly iron and calcium. The more varied the DIET, the greater the chance of including all the required MINERALS and VITAMINS.

● Eating extra dairy products is not the best way to increase a pregnant woman's calcium intake. Drinking twice as much milk can upset the digestive system and add weight. An abundance of calcium is available in cabbage, turnip greens, spinach, broccoli, kale, parsnips. Nuts, pulses, raw oats and whole

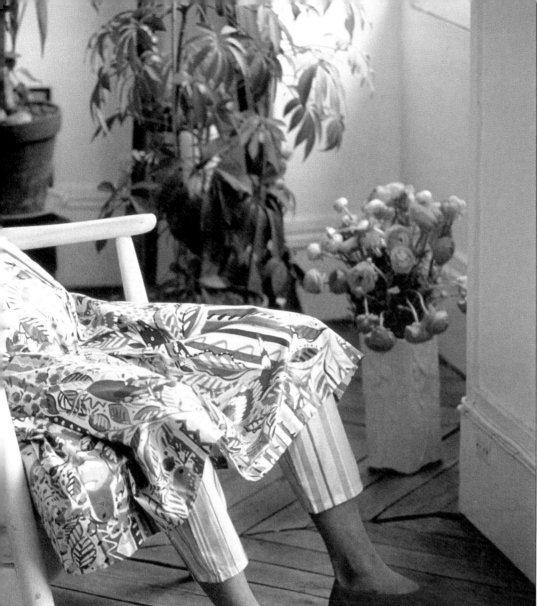

SEX
Lovemaking is extra special during pregnancy and there's no reason why it should stop. You will need to experiment with positions as you get larger. But as long as you feel good about it and there is no discomfort, there is no reason why you should stop making love.

WORK
Still working? That's up to you. Listen to your body. If you are feeling fit and well, there's no reason you shouldn't continue working until the birth. There are no hard and fast rules. If you have to work because money is scarce, make sure you get enough rest in the evening and realise your own limitations. You'll be surprised how sympathetic fellow workers can be if you need to rest during the day. Pregnancy involves common sense and listening to what your body and baby tell you.

YOU
You're special, so give yourself treats. Go shopping for new maternity clothes to fit the new, expanding you. Have your hair restyled into an easier-to-look-after shape. Make time to see friends and relatives – people you enjoy being with. Honour yourself, buy flowers. How about new underwear for the creative you!

EMOTIONS
A mother's psychological state is now believed to have a direct influence on the foetus. An increase in foetal heart rate accompanies maternal anxiety. If this is prolonged and severe it may cause distress to the unborn child.

P

grains contain smaller amounts, and, to a lesser extent, rhubarb, dates, apricots, raisins, oranges, prunes, peaches and figs are also sources of calcium.

● Try to avoid iron in tablet form, as it can increase constipation. Eat plenty of iron-rich foods instead – good sources include liver, free-range eggs, dairy produce, watercress, dried apricots, wholewheat bread, cocoa and carob, cabbage, alfalfa, beetroot, cherries, sunflower seeds, blackcurrants, blackberries, lentils. Vitamin C enhances iron absorption so keep peeling those citrus fruits!

● Zinc is essential for the healthy growth of the foetus. Good sources of zinc are meats, liver, cheese, wheatgerm, whole grains, nuts, green beans and lima beans.

● Ruthlessly cut out fatteners like sweets, cakes, chocolates. They are

not doing either of you any good.

BACK CARE
● High levels of the hormone progesterone soften tendons and ligaments to accommodate the growing baby. Be aware of posture, and bad sitting position.

EXERCISE
● If you exercise regularly before pregnancy, it will be safe for you to continue to do so until it feels uncomfortable. Accept that you may need to slow down during the later stages of pregnancy. If you want to take up an exercise during pregnancy, swimming is the safest. Take it easy. The water bears your weight and all major muscles are used.

Check locally to find out about special ante-natal exercise classes in your area.

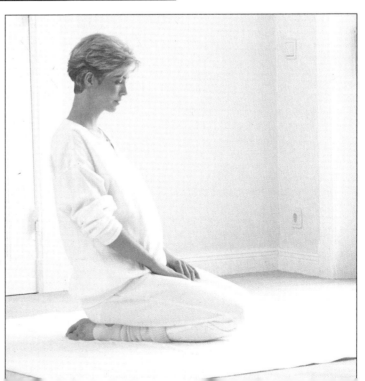

Taking up meditation or learning relaxation techniques during pregnancy is a good idea.

(See EMOTIONS, COUNSELLING, MEDITATION, YOGA, AUTOGENICS, BIOFEEDBACK.)

LOVING WAYS

Love is as important as health. A mother who feels and shows joy towards her developing child by lovingly massaging her abdomen and by speaking in soothing and welcoming tones to it will give birth to a child who has no doubts about its right to exist. Cradled for protection inside the womb, it is secure in the knowledge that it is loved and wanted.

And that is the greatest gift any parent can give.

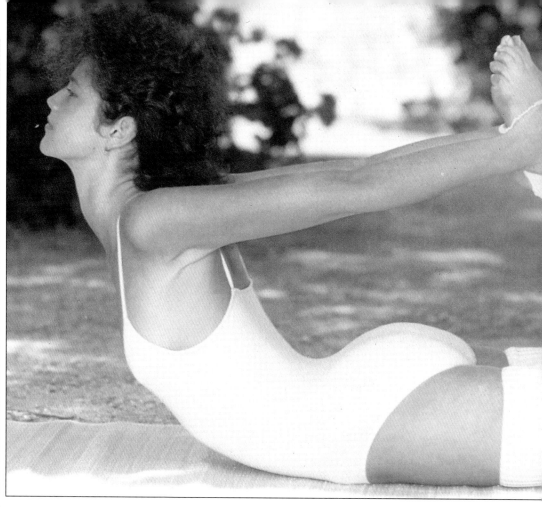

PREMENSTRUAL SYNDROME

Premenstrual syndrome refers to a variety of symptoms experienced only in the week to ten days before a period is due.

In some cases this can extend to half the entire menstrual cycle, beginning at mid-cycle when ovulation takes place and continuing until the next period.

PMS has many physical symptoms including fluid retention, tender breasts, abdominal bloating, back pain, fatigue, headaches and nausea. Many women experience depression or weepiness, irritability, loss of concentration, while some become violent, exhibiting dramatic personality changes.

There is a positive side to PMS. Some women describe an enhancement of creativity and perceptiveness and a richness of imagery and imagination – responses are heightened.

Being premenstrual is not an illness. It's likely that changes in the activity of the body's control centre – the hypothalamus – cause an imbalance during part of the menstrual cycle. The hypothalamus is involved directly and indirectly with the production of certain hormones and stimulates the nervous system. To believe that the body is out of kilter for a while is different from believing that parts of your body are diseased or breaking down. It helps to be positive and say to yourself while suffering PMS symptoms, 'I usually have a healthy body, but the balance of it changes for part of the month.'

PMS can be used positively to question certain areas of your life and to change them. Tensions in relationships, smoking, poor diet, stress are some of the many factors which may trigger a change of activity in the hypothalamus, and which certainly exacerbate PMS. Women who try to positively change some aspects of their lives, or develop skills such as relaxation to counter PMS, begin to feel in control – no longer victims of PMS, but managers of it.

Here are some pointers to help ease PMS symptoms. . .

Remove all refined starches, processed foods and additives from your diet. Reduce sugar, tea, coffee and alcohol intake and eat more fresh fruit and vegetables.

Vitamin B6 has been found to help symptoms of depression and bloating. It should be taken as a supplement with other B vitamins and instructions for dosage carefully followed.

Supplements of magnesium and calcium are traditionally used to treat premenstrual and menstrual cramps.

Fatigue can be caused by low potassium. Do not take as a supplement – high concentrations of potassium can cause heart problems – but increase through diet. Eat plenty of nuts, fresh fruit and vegetables, grains, fruits, KELP and garlic.

EVENING PRIMROSE OIL is effective for breast tenderness and swelling and can help emotional symptoms. (The exact dosage for PMS has not yet been established. It is usually prepared in capsules of 0.5 grams to be taken three to four times daily throughout the month. Try this dosage for one month and if it is not successful, increase capsules to six a day. If necessary, increase to eight on the third month. After that reduce until you are able to take one a day.) Always take with food.

Progesterone therapy can relieve emotional symptoms. It is taken sublingually (under the tongue), as suppository or by injection. It is not to be confused with the progesterone-like substances (progestogens) that are used in birth control pills. There can be side effects such as irregular spotting, cramps and diarrhoea.

Beat stress by learning relaxation skills. Join an evening class in yoga or any other form of meditation.

Acupuncture, chiropractic, aromatherapy and massage are all effective therapies for PMS.

Join or start up a PMS support group. Share your PMS experiences with women friends. Isolation can make matters worse.

(See ACUPUNCTURE, CHIROPRACTIC, MASSAGE, MEDITATION, MENSTRUATION, YOGA.)

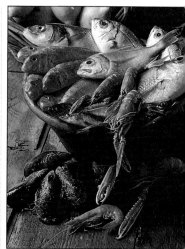

PROTEIN

Protein means 'of prime importance' and makes up 17 per cent of our body weight. It is used in the structure of our bones, skin, hair and muscle and contributes to enzyme and hormone production, including insulin which controls the body's blood sugar levels.

The building blocks of protein are called AMINO ACIDS. Foods such as fish and other seafoods, lean meat, cheese, eggs, yoghurt and milk are

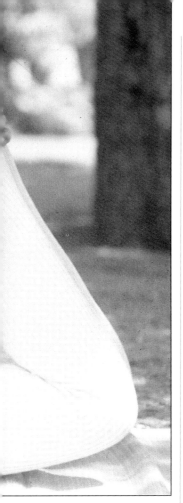

high in protein. Vegetable foods with a reasonably high protein content include beans, peas, lentils, nuts, seeds, grain and soya products such as tofu. Department of Health recommends an average daily protein intake of 69 grams a day for men and 54 grams for women – representing 10% of energy intake.

PULSE

The strength of the heart is reflected by your pulse rate. A strong heart may need to beat only 60 times or less in a minute to keep the blood flowing around the body. To take your pulse rate place three fingers of one hand on the underside of the opposite wrist until you feel a throb. Count your pulse for 30 seconds and then multiply by two for rate per minute. Do this before getting up in the morning.

The average resting pulse rate is about 70 beats per minute, but it can vary from 50 to 100, depending on health. Use your resting pulse to gauge your fitness. Take your pulse rate repeatedly five seconds after exercising – the quicker it returns to its resting rate the fitter you are.

Qi

Qi is an ancient Chinese medical tradition with which acupuncture, acupressure and herbal remedies are all connected. Qi means vital energy, the very force which keeps us alive. It is believed to flow through specific conduits of the meridians. (See ACUPUNCTURE.)

Qi is divided into three categories: original Qi is transmitted from parents and is finite, as it is used little by little over time; nutritional Qi is extracted from the food we eat and is constantly utilised from the air you breathe. An imbalance of Qi is believed to cause ill health.

Qi Gong is a form of martial art. It combines deep, controlled exercise, physical training and intense concentration which directs Qi to certain parts of the body.

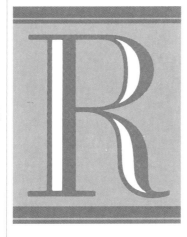

REFLEXOLOGY

Reflexology is the therapy in which the reflexes in the feet are believed to correspond with every part of the body via ten 'energy paths' running between the feet and head.

Using mainly thumbs and index fingers, the reflexologist seeks out tender areas and from these can identify problems in other parts of the body. Reflexology can help bring about normal functioning of all the organs and glands, improve nerve function and circulation and induce a state of relaxation. It also aids lymphatic and venous circulation and can help migraines, sinusitis and digestive problems.

Two 40-minute visits a week for three weeks are generally recommended, but up to 30 visits may be necessary for full benefit. This therapy is often used in conjunction with aromatherapy, herbalism, massage and naturopathy.

RELAXATION

You are walking through a cool, green forest. There's a glimpse of the sea sparkling in the sunlight between the branches. The perfume of warm pine fills your head and as you walk along the scented pathway you have a wonderful feeling of liberation and peace.

You may not want to walk through a forest, you might prefer being massaged with warm oil giving you a lovely all-over feeling of warmth, or splash through a tropical sea. Once you've learned simple relaxation techniques, there's no end to the wonderful places you can visit and the warm, self-healing feeling you can experience. Your first step is to learn simple relaxation techniques. There are several ways you can do this, through AUTOGENICS, BIOFEEDBACK, MEDITATION, YOGA, or by listening to relaxation tapes. It may take several attempts, but don't be discouraged.

Relaxation is an essential skill for anyone wishing to counter the effects of STRESS and anxiety in their life. Once mastered and put to regular use, the benefits and pleasure of deep relaxation are considerable. It lowers blood pressure, controls psychosomatic problems such as asthma, increases energy levels, alleviates menstrual tension, enhances dream recall and creativity and improves health generally. You can alter the sequence and details of relaxation techniques to suit you.

Put aside 20 minutes a day for two weeks to concentrate on the following basic steps to relaxation and incorporate it into your daily routine. If you prefer, get a friend to guide you through the steps initially, or make a tape to guide you.

● Lie comfortably, cover yourself

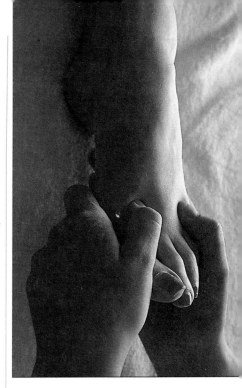

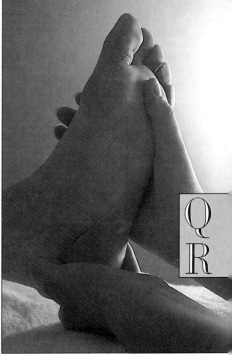

with a blanket and select a point on the ceiling above you.

● Stare at the point without blinking. Remind your body what it feels like to go to sleep – visualise your limbs being heavy and warm. You are sinking and floating.

● Keep focusing on that spot on the ceiling, and feel your eyes slowly closing. Embrace the warm sleepy darkness in your head and body.

● Be aware of the big toe on your left foot. Don't move it. Just know it is there, sense the space it occupies, its warmth. Move to your right toe then

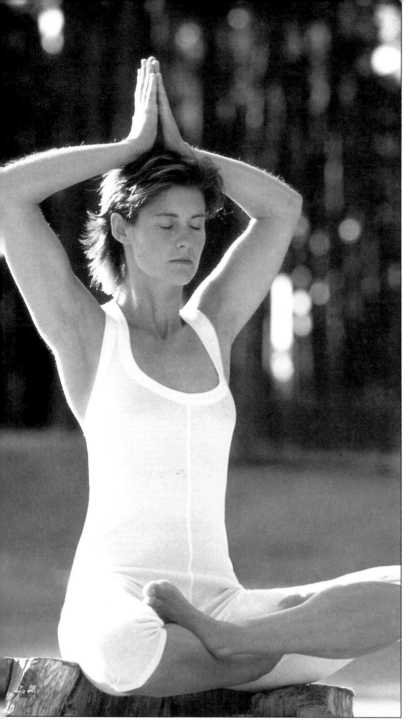

for example. Imagine the colours, feel the softness of the petals, breathe in the heady mix of perfumes. Stay in this pleasant place for as long as you need to.

● When you are ready, imagine you are a diver returning from great depths to the light playing above the water. Count backwards from 20 as you do so. Open your eyes when you reach number one.

● Move very gently at first, and don't rush anywhere. Spend time savouring the feeling of refreshment and revitalisation. When you are ready, go out and meet the world. You have a sanctuary that's all your own, where you can feel at peace, and which takes you away from the stress and rush of the outside world. Use it.

ROLFING

Rolfing is a method of manipulating the connective tissues of the body in order to realign the structure. Its practitioners aim to increase range of movement, improve balance and promote better posture.

The Rolfing technique is a mixture of osteopathy and massage. Rolfers use their fingers and sometimes elbows to move and stretch muscles, tissues and ligaments to help regain their elasticity and full range of movement. A course usually comprises ten weekly sessions. Photographs are taken during the treatment so that the client can see the improvements in posture and balance that have been made.

The largest group of people to benefit from Rolfing have chronic pain related to the body's soft tissue structure, such as non-inflammatory arthritis, stiff joints or back pain. Whiplash injuries also respond well, as do some sports injuries, including jogger's knee and tennis elbow.

ROYAL JELLY

Worker bees produce royal jelly for their queen by secreting a milky-white, gelatinous substance from their salivary glands. Research shows that royal jelly is highly nutritious and can support the body's immune system. It is also believed to protect against leukaemia and treat bone disorders such as rheumatoid arthritis.

Many pregnant women and mothers who are breast-feeding take royal jelly. As in all cases where pregnancy is concerned, a doctor should be consulted first.

allow this focused awareness to spread through to your other toes, soles, heels and slowly the whole foot. Feel how warm and heavy your feet are getting.

Let this relaxing, melting feeling spread up the rest of the leg as you focus on each part – the shins, the calves, the knees, the thighs.

Let the warmth of relaxation run up your back and caress each part of your body until it runs like warm oil over your chest, moves like warm soft hands on to your shoulder blades, softens your neck and soothes the chin.

● Feel your breathing come and go as it will. It is the link between the conscious and the unconscious.

● Start to concentrate on the outbreath. Feel yourself relaxing each time you breathe out. Imagine you are breathing out from an inch or two above your navel. Your body feels as though it is gently opening out like a flower.

Allow any thoughts or dream pictures to come, look at them, let them go. This is the place you can draw on images of your own making, walking in a forest or relaxing on a tropical beach.

Be where you would most like to be – in a beautiful country garden,

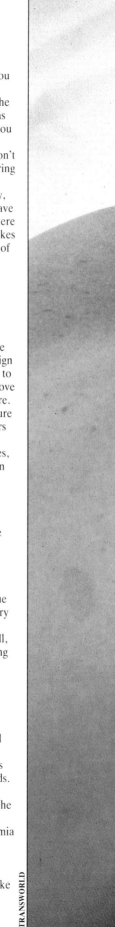

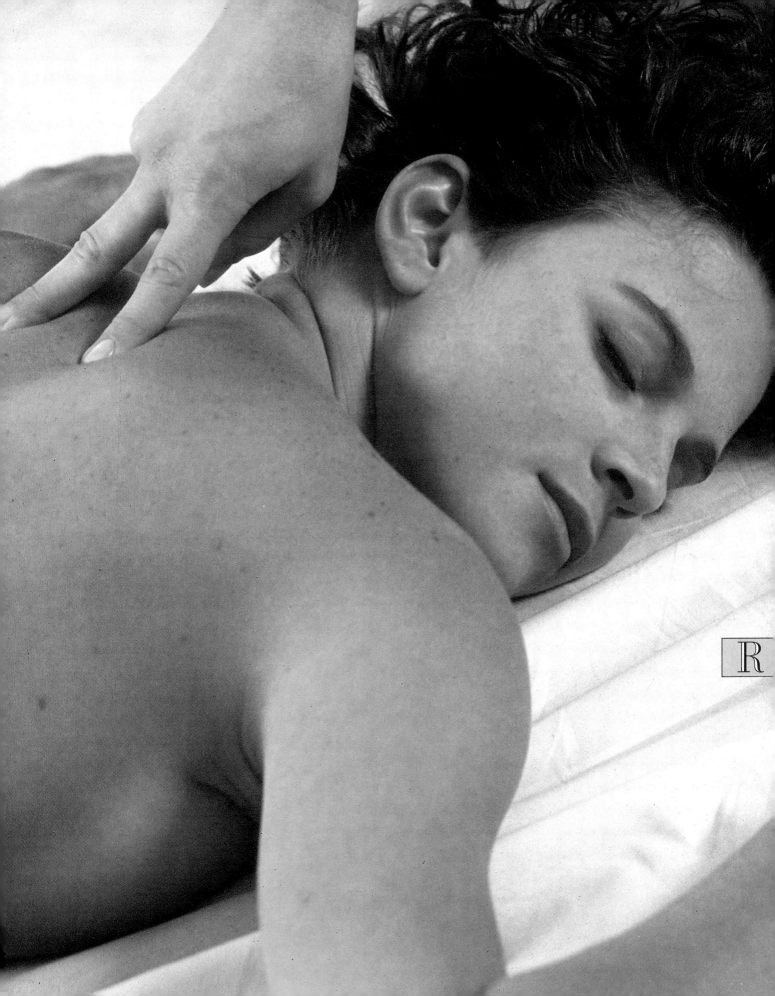

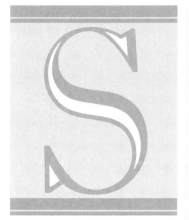

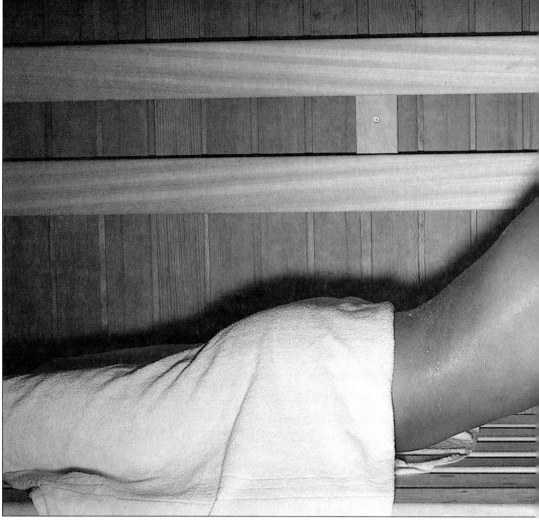

SAUNA

Saunas make you sweat – that's the intention. For centuries sweating has been seen as a healthy way to cleanse the body of toxins, stimulate circulation and rejuvenate. In today's sedentary and air-cooled conditions, the trouble is that we don't sweat as much as we should. Our perspiration-linked purification system isn't used to full capacity. Saunas can help us out.

All that sweating causes fluid loss. The body uses up three calories for each teaspoon of water lost. The body loses approximately two quarts of water in one hour of heavy sweating. Ten to 15 minutes in a sauna could burn up 100 to 200 calories. That might not sound much, but while you're just lying there, the calories lost are equal to the number you would lose by a mile of walking.

When you sit in the sauna you are putting your body under the same stress as exercise, but this time it's responding to heat. Your body works to keep cool – breathing becomes heavier, the heart beats faster, the pulse feels stronger, and the blood vessels in the skin expand in the effort to get the heat out. Like some exercise, sweat bathing – whether it's a Turkish bath or sauna – gets your heart and lungs working. (And that is why anyone with diabetes, high blood pressure or a heart condition should seek medical advice before having a sauna.)

Sweating it out improves skin, too. But never spend more than ten minutes at a time in a sauna. Follow up with a brief, coldish shower, relax and repeat sauna–shower routine if you want to. Always end with a brisk rub down with a towel or loofah and then moisturise all over. Saunas can ease menstrual cramps and helps eliminate retained water.

SAUNA TIPS
Take it easy first few times. Spend five minutes on lower bench where it's cooler
Gradually increase the time you spend in the sauna, using comfort level as guide
As soon as you feel uncomfortable get out
Don't eat a big meal before hand, or drink alcohol, tea or coffee

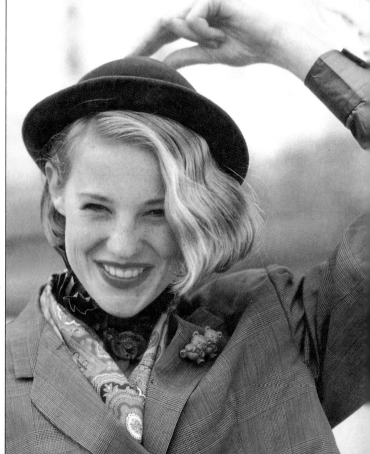

SELF-ESTEEM

Crucial to emotional and mental well-being is self-esteem. The foundation of self-esteem lies in having a strong sense of self, which comes from within and is not dependent on the goodwill of others. If your sense of self-worth depends on friends, family, colleagues or partners, you will be reluctant to jeopardise it and you'll find yourself doing things you don't want to do, agreeing when you disagree and repressing negative feelings.

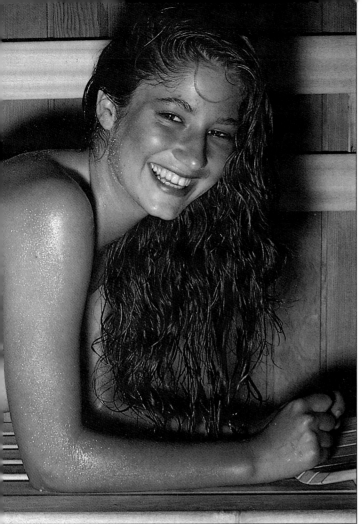

increases. There's a sudden boost in secretion of the sex hormones oestrogen, progesterone, androgen and testosterone. It's likely that this hormonal increase is responsible for the higher red blood cell count and improved circulation in sexually active men and women. Muscles in the thighs, tummy and buttocks are exercised, burning up an average of 200 calories and expending the equivalent amount of energy used to run two miles.

A fulfilling sex life can improve your diet, too. According to psychologists, sex can help reduce craving for comfort foods such as sugar, sweets and alcohol – all high in calories. So avoid the temptation of post-coital snacks! Those hunger pangs are caused by a drop in blood sugar levels which can be raised with glucose tablets.

Like any regular exercise, sex fights stress. Sleep after lovemaking is deep and refreshing and all that touching,

HOT AND SPICY
Essential oils for erotic massage
For her:
Pimento berry is spicy and passionate, wild and vivid
Rose bulgar is like silk stroking the skin
Clary–sage is heady and euphoric
For him:
Myrrh is musky and smoky, mysteriously seductive
Cardamom is sensuously spicy
Jasmine seduces
Mace is warm, soft and sultry

stroking and kissing has the same therapeutic value as massage. Love not only makes the world go round, it helps you live longer and suffer less from colds and flu.

A poor diet, alcohol, ill health, and stress and lack of communication will dilute passion. A combination of safe sex and a fit body increases alertness, enhances mental faculties and puts a

Developing self-esteem means. . .
- Valuing yourself for who you are.
- Knowing your limitations.
- Appreciating others for who they are, not for what you want them to be.
- Trusting your own judgment without constantly referring to an outside authority.

You are more likely to have a positive self-image if you had a loving, secure childhood with parents who also had a good sense of themselves. If low self-esteem results from childhood experiences, you may need professional help from a counsellor or psychotherapist to build up feelings of self-worth. (See COUNSELLING).

Here's a start in building a strong sense of self. . .
- Define clearly what you want out of life.
- Aim high, imagining how you would like to live – think about what makes you happiest.
- Write down your personal goals – they help to focus and direct your energy and give a sense of purpose and self-reliance.
- Listen to your inner voice through meditation or other relaxation techniques. (See MEDITATION.

RELAXATION.)
- Be honest with yourself and others.
- Take responsibility for yourself and your actions; don't blame others.
- Don't constantly seek the approval of others – especially parents. It stops you meeting your own needs and hinders self-respect.

S^{EX}

Sex does wonders for health and beauty – it comes tops in the exercise stakes. At its best it tones muscles, beats stress, is a powerful relaxant and energises.

At the first touch, eyes start to shine and pupils begin to dilate. As excitement mounts, breasts increase in size and pectoral muscles start to twitch slightly. The side walls of the nose expand slightly, widening nostrils. Breathing deepens, bringing more oxygen into the body and producing that heady sensation associated with passion.

The body's temperature increases by two to three degrees, blood pressure rises slightly and circulation

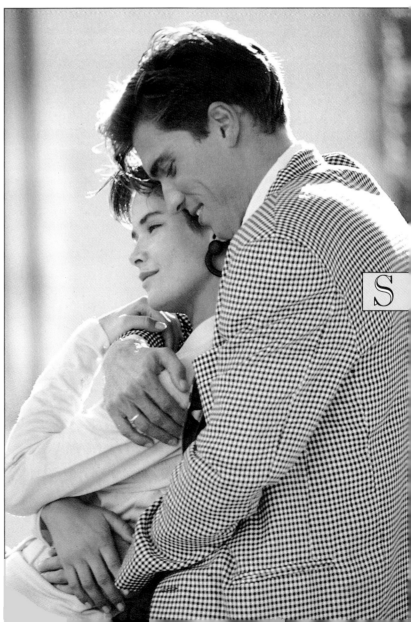

S

twinkle in the eye. For exercises to give your sex life a boost, see SEXERCISE.

SAFE SEX

The key to safe sex and preventing transfer of HIV is not just a question of how often you have sex and how many sexual partners you have. It's the *way* you have sex.

Aids presents us with some basic challenges about the way we live our lives and express our sexuality, and we may find ourselves enriched by the experience. Suddenly we all have to be *sure* that we are living our sexual lives with responsibility, care and respect for ourselves and others. Safer sex isn't a denial of our sexuality. Safe sex can be better sex.

The main obstacle to safe sex is our sexual conditioning. 'Real' sex is usually seen exclusively as penetrative intercourse. Other forms of sexual expression tend to be seen as a preparation for penetration. But penetration is not essential for sexual satisfaction, as most women know. Surveys show that women are least likely to come to orgasm during penetration and that men often prefer to be stimulated to orgasm by other means.

Safe sex is an opportunity to discover erogenous zones you never thought you had and explore to the full your sexual potential. Caressing, hugging and cuddling break down the barriers of distance, introduce the magic of touch and create feelings of warmth and security.

Massage each other with your own

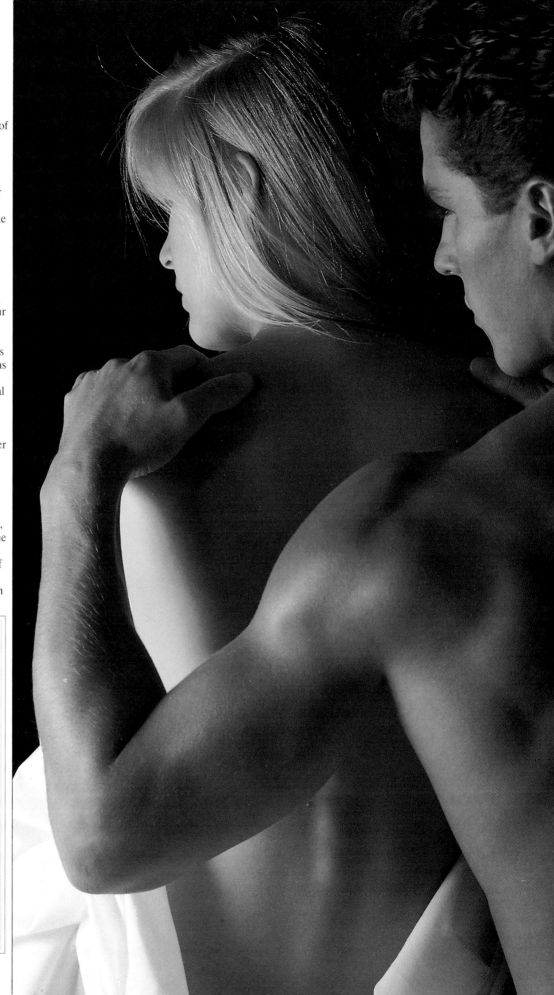

PLAYING SAFELY
You can have a lot of fun with…
Caressing, hugging, cuddling
Massage
Body kissing
Mutual masturbation
Body to body rubbing

A condom must be used for intercourse if you are unsure of your partner's history and care taken that the condom does not come off or split. Spermicides containing nonoxynol (such as Duragel, Orthocreme or Delfen cream) may offer added protection. All lubricants used with a condom should be water-based (KY and 1-2-1); grease-based lubricants such as Vaseline, baby oil etc rapidly damage the rubber of the condom so that it stops offering protection
Avoid any sexual practice that draws blood or breaks the skin

potent mixture of super-sexy essential oils (see previous page) using six drops to 15ml (½oz) vegetable oil – almond, soya, peanut, hazelnut or peach kernel. Massage gently into the skin all over, lingering where your partner says it feels best.

Body kissing

The mouth and tongue are exquisitely sensitive organs and, in combination with the sensuality of skin, present endless possibilities – licking, sucking, nuzzling, and especially kissing. Like music, kissing has moods, tones and rhythms that can create a repertoire of sensations and responses. Natural body tastes can be a turn-on too, or create your own with strawberries, honey, champagne.

Lights-off and under-the-blanket sex ignores the erotic potential of the sense of sight. It's easy to forget how important a part it plays in our sexual lives, from admiring and enjoying our bodies to looking at another's. Visually enjoying your partner's body is a powerful aphrodisiac.

Erogenous ears

How about 'talking dirty'? Your ears are erogenous zones in more ways than one. Listening to your own and your partner's sounds of delight can enhance pleasure, and background music can be a powerful erotic stimulus.

Sexual fantasies are normal and we all have them. Exchange your favourite most erotic fantasies with your lover. But give it a miss if either partner finds the other's fantasies distressing, threatening, or arouse jealousy. Personal sharing on this level needs to be treated with respect.

Consider and talk about the kinds of loveplay you and your partner enjoy best – dressing up, undressing, baths and showers, masturbation, cuddling, sexy underwear, role playing, sensual oils, telephone calls . . . the possibilities for safe sex are fun and endless.

Abstinence is, of course, the safest choice for many people, but that needn't mean a life without love or romance.

IAN BRADSHAW, STEVE SHIPMAN

SEXERCISE

Lovemaking is an exhilarating exercise in its own right, but to enjoy its full potential you need to be supple and relaxed. There are certain exercises that can increase muscle power and stamina for both men and women. (Consult your doctor before doing these exercises if you have back problems.) Try these two in bed:

 Lie on your right side, curl up in a ball and hug your knees.
 Stretch out, arms above head, toes pointed.
 Curl up again.
 Roll over to left side, stretch, curl, and repeat five times.

Good for the back, tummy and posture.

Still in bed. . .
 Remove pillows, lie on tummy with hands at sides and your head flat to one side.
 Raise left leg as high as possible, cross over right leg and gently lower.
 Repeat with right leg.
Repeat exercise five times.

Rocking pelvis – designed to loosen the lower back area, combining deep breathing with thrusting pelvic movements.
 Lie on your back on the floor.
 As you breathe in, rock pelvis slowly backwards by arching the small of your back.
 As you breathe out, tilt your pelvis upwards, pushing the small of your back against the floor.

It may help to have your hands on your hips as you are practising the motion.

Try for two minutes at first and build up to five minutes. Don't hurry and try to co-ordinate breathing with pelvic movement.

Bouncing pelvis – heightens awareness of pelvic feelings.
 Lie on back with knees up.
 Raise hips and bounce pelvis up and down.
 Use hands to raise your body if necessary and bounce for one minute, building up to three minutes.

Combining any of the above with half an hour of walking, swimming, cycling or running at least three times a week will enhance your love life. For women, any of the antenatal exercises which strengthen the pelvic floor are good for sex. Also try deep BREATHING exercises as a relaxant.

SHIATSU

In shiatsu, disease is seen as blocked and unbalanced energy. It is either depleted (kyo) or overactive (jitsu). Illness is manifest as jitsu on the surface but its cause is believed to lie with kyo – deep-seated and hidden.

Using the palms, fingers, thumb, knuckles, elbows and even feet, the shiatsu practitioner works on the hundreds of ACUPUNCTURE points (tsubos) along the body's meridians

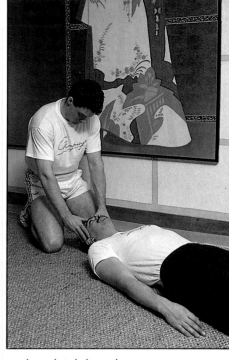

or channels to balance the energy flow that maintains health and vitality. Shiatsu developed from the ancient Japanese massage called amna, which involved rubbing the hands and feet with the fingers and palms of the hands. It is probably rooted in our natural response to pain – to 'rub it better' when hurt. It shares with traditional Chinese medicine the belief that all phenomena are divided into two complementary energy forces; Yin, the negative, and Yang the positive.

Shiatsu can effectively treat stress-related disorder and everyday ailments, and can reduce pain in childbirth. During or after treatment you may experience a variety of reactions as the energy in your body shifts and balances. Feelings of intense sadness, tears, laughter, joy, or slight discomfort are all positive signs that shiatsu is working for you.

If you decide to try a shiatsu massage, make sure you find a properly qualified practitioner. You have to be qualified in massage before you can train in shiatsu, but you might like to try some of the simpler shiatsu techniques on yourself. . .
 Apply the pressure as you breathe out, because this is the time when you are most relaxed.
 Use thumb or palm pressure as these are easily controlled.
 For insomnia, press with thumb for ten seconds on tsubo one finger's width to the side of the eyebrow between the end of the eyebrow and the outer edge of eye.
 For stress headaches, press your thumbs on nape of neck at base of the skull for seven to ten seconds, three times.

SKIN

The skin your body wears is approximately 18 feet square, and weighs ten pounds. It protects your body from heat and cold, the elements and bacteria. It's waterproof, elastic and versatile. The skin's surface (epidermis) is made up of dead cells – new cells grow from the bottom layer of the epidermis to the outside in approximately three weeks, then they drop off.

Beneath the epidermis, another layer, the dermis, is full of fat cells, hair follicles and glands pumping out sweat and other fluids including pheromones – which are supposed to attract the opposite sex. The sebaceous glands pump out sebum which protects and oils the skin. Nerves and blood vessels carry messages, supply food and oxygen to all the active parts of the skin. The rich supply of sensory nerve endings on the skin's surface relay the whole range of sensations of touch to the brain – from sensual to painful.

The colour of your skin reflects the history of evolution, as people over the ages have adapted to different environments.

Black skin has greater protection against sunburn, and tends to age less quickly than white skin. When early humans travelled north from Africa, skins became pale to prevent vitamin D deficiency from lack of sun.

Skin accurately reflects your state of health. A glowing, vibrant skin that functions efficiently depends on a healthy balanced DIET, plenty of EXERCISE and loving care. Remember your skin is under constant stress – from the weather, extremes of temperature, environmental pollution, household chemicals – and it needs constant pampering. Get to know its enemies and become your skin's best friend.

Dehydration: central heating, air conditioning, air travel, alcohol and hormonal changes all rob the skin of its moisture. Drink plenty of water – it's the main ingredient for a soft, youthful-looking skin. Both men and women should apply plenty of moisturiser – all over after a bath or shower, and on the face and hands during the day and before going to bed at night. For dry skin take regular doses of EVENING PRIMROSE OIL until condition clears.

Poor waste elimination: if the major elimination organs such as the kidneys, colon and lymphatic system aren't functioning efficiently, a variety of skin diseases including eczema and boils can erupt as the body tries to push more toxins through the skin than it can cope with. Drink plenty of water, cut down on alcohol and give junk food a miss. If you're regularly constipated, eat more fibre and drink several cups of fennel tea daily (see HERBALISM). A glass of warm water with the juice of a squeezed lemon before breakfast every morning helps, too.

Sunshine: too much sun can rapidly age skin and cause skin cancer. Experts advise applying a sun protection cream all year round – including winter – to neutralise the damaging effects of the sun's ULTRAVIOLET RAYS.

Smoking: oxygen is essential for healthy skin. Smoking not only reduces amounts of oxygen used by the blood, but slows down its supply. Skin becomes sallow and lifeless, and lines appear around the mouth.

Allergies: very often allergies to specific foods can be first detected on your skin as irritating spots, rashes or eczema. (See ALLERGIES.)

Neglect: skin can suffer from lack of touch. Develop a flair for MASSAGE with your partner. Use the fragrant and healing powers of essential oils to soothe and enrich the skin. Spoil yourself! Visit an aromatherapist every month. Regular lovemaking adds glow and sparkle to skin, too. (See SEX.)

Every day give your skin the first class treatment it deserves. Wash or,

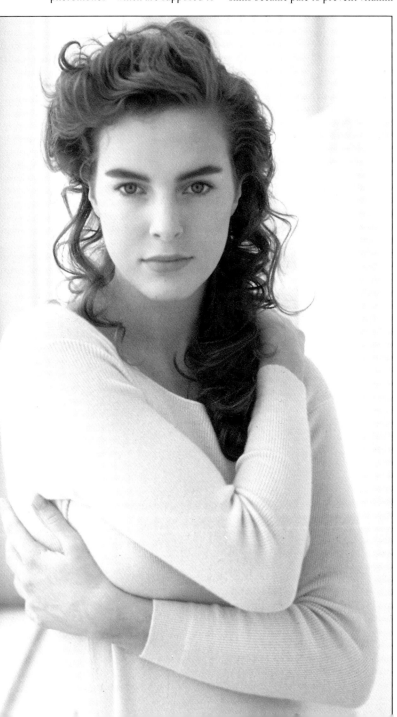

if you wear make-up or work in a city, use cleansing oil or cream cleanser, then splash with cold water. In the bath or shower use a loofah all over to slough off dead cells and stimulate circulation, or rub gently with an exfoliating scrub. Splash with cold water to close pores, then moisturise.

SLEEP

A good sleep regenerates the body, strengthens the IMMUNE SYSTEM, repairs damaged tissues and cells and helps relax you mentally.

Although we spend a third of our lives sleeping, relatively little is known about it. Some people require more sleep than others, but the amount of sleep is not the most important factor, it's the quality that counts.

An average night's sleep has a series of four or five cycles, each lasting between one to two hours and

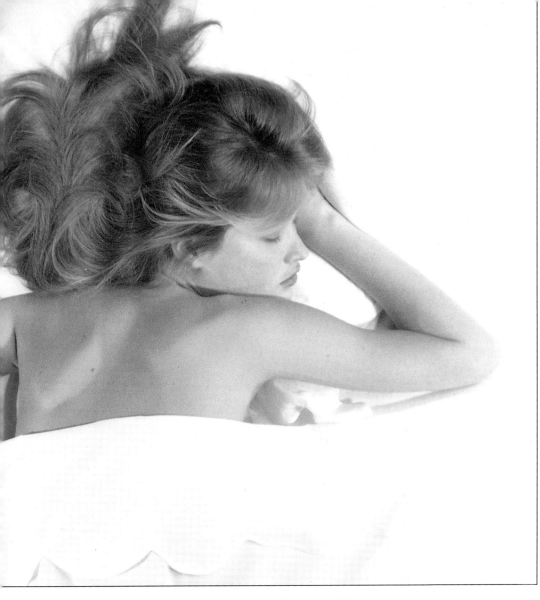

made up of five stages. The first four stages in each cycle are known as orthodox sleep and the fifth is referred to as 'dream sleep'.

During the first stages of orthodox sleep brain waves slow down and bodily functions such as blood pressure decrease. Hormone production from the pituitary gland increases, regenerating the entire body. In the fifth stage, dreaming occurs with rapid eye movement (REM). It is this phase of sleep which is thought to be essential for our emotional and mental equilibrium.

The Ancient Greeks used dreams to heal and prophesy. Sigmund Freud pioneered dream study in the 20th century, seeing dreams as the gateway to understanding the unconscious mind. More recent research has produced the theory that dreams help us practise our learned behaviour – integrating new information with the knowledge we already have each night.

While you are dreaming you look completely relaxed, but your body is working hard. Breathing returns to its normal daily rate, blood pressure and temperature rise and adrenalin rockets into the system. Your eyes move rapidly in their sockets – you are watching your dreams just as you would a cinema film or television. Dreams occur regularly throughout the night, usually lasting no more than ten minutes, but often culminating in a half hour epic just before you wake up.

To ensure a good night's sleep:

Forget that bedtime mug of cocoa – its caffeine content stimulates in the same way tea, coffee and alcohol do. Drink a relaxing cup of herb tea instead – try camomile, lemon verbena or passion flower. (See HERBALISM.)

Don't eat a heavy meal before sleeping.

Exercising before bedtime lifts energy and leaves you wide awake; a winding down routine is better.

Sleeping problems? See INSOMNIA.

SMOKING

Nicotine is as addictive as heroin. Its hooks go deep, involving complex physiological and psychological mechanisms that drive and maintain the smoker.

Like heroin, nicotine is an alkaloid found in plants. The alkaloid kills insects by disrupting their neurotransmitters – substances released by the bugs' activated nerve cells. Humans have the same neurotransmitters. But what is toxic to a bug is pleasurable to the human when taken in the small amounts contained in cigarettes. Heroin attaches itself to the natural painkilling receptors, but nicotine affects the major neurotransmitter system which conducts nerve signals, memory and their critical functions. Once in the body it is carried within seconds to most body tissues by binding itself to white blood cells.

But nicotine differs from other addictive drugs in several ways:

Its effects are felt more rapidly than drugs taken intravenously. One quarter of the nicotine in each drag reaches the brain in seven seconds. The nicotine concentration in the blood peaks at about the time the cigarette butt is extinguished. The effects fall off rapidly as the nicotine is cleared by the liver and excreted in the urine.

Within half an hour most smokers are reaching for another cigarette. A pack-a-day smoker takes 70,000 drug 'hits' a year.

Nicotine does not interfere with normal activity.

The smoker uses nicotine to fine-tune the body's reactions to the world and is incredibly adept at maintaining a steady concentration of nicotine in the bloodstream throughout the day. There is an internal sensing system, something like a heating thermostat, which knows when nicotine levels are too low. It prompts a smoker to light up when the nicotine level needs

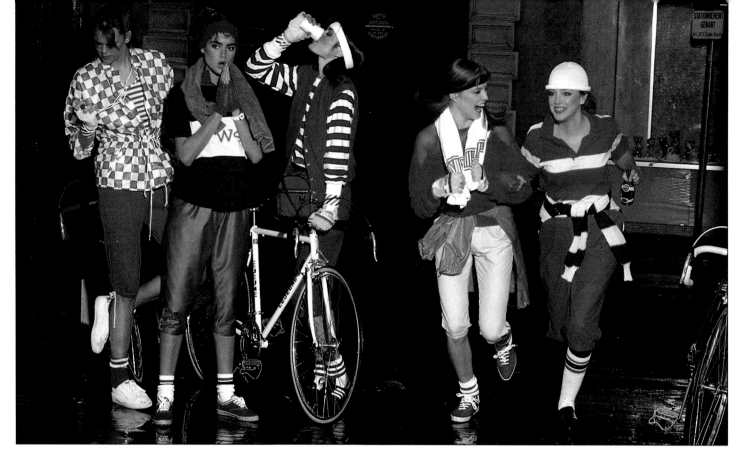

boosting. Most smokers need a minimum of ten cigarettes to maintain a comfortable threshold. Watch a cigarette addict drawing on his first cigarette of the day. He will inhale the smoke deeply to lift fallen nicotine levels.

Nicotine improves short-term memory and gives subjective relief from stress, while at the same time inducing the biological symptoms of stress by speeding up the heart rate and raising blood pressure. A smoker's heartbeat is increased about eight to ten beats a minute all day and night – producing excessive wear on the heart. It's not only the nicotine in

THE HARD FACTS OF SMOKING
Smoking kills over 100,000 people in the UK each year
In 1987, 44,546 people died of heart disease directly caused by smoking
Approximately 36,000 people die from lung cancer and a further 25,714 people die from bronchitis and emphysema caused by smoking
Women smokers are three and a half times more likely to suffer cervical cancer
Smoking is implicated in male and female infertility
Smokers give birth to babies that are usually 200g smaller than average and remain underweight until early adulthood

a cigarette that causes trouble, but everything else that goes with it – the tar, the carbon monoxide and thousands of poisons that find their way into the lungs and then around the body – which can also contribute to life-threatening problems, such as heart and lung disease.

Research shows that nicotine withdrawal symptoms include anxiety, irritability, lack of concentration, cravings, drowsiness, decreased heart rate, tremors and slowed metabolism. The smoker who wants to kick the habit needs a great deal of support and will only succeed, say the experts, if he or she really *wants* to. Feeling that you *ought* to isn't reason enough.

There are new developments on the give-up-smoking horizon. Drugs used to treat people with opiate withdrawal have been shown to block some of the effects of nicotine and are being used experimentally at the moment to help people stop smoking.

Replacement therapies satisfy the smoker's dependence on nicotine while he or she unlearns the psychological habits that drive smoking behaviour. They have tended to be in the form of gum that can be chewed, but a nicotine nose spray and a skin patch which releases nicotine slowly into the blood are now being tested.

A nicotine substitute, Nicobrevin, is also available. Taken in capsule

form, it contains quinine, a natural sedative, and eucalyptus.

It is best to avoid nicotine supplements and use other methods which can help just as effectively and don't continue to expose your body to the effects of nicotine. HYPNOSIS. ACUPUNCTURE and aversion therapy have all helped smokers to give up successfully.

Once you've decided to give up smoking, make sure you enlist the support and understanding of those close to you. After all, they are going to have to bear the brunt of your withdrawal symptoms. They need to be sympathetically involved.

SPORT

Sport is a fun way to exercise. It can enhance your social life – team members can become new friends. Team ball games such as football, netball and basketball can help you improve co-ordination and, depending on the position you play, can be AEROBIC – you need to be moving constantly for approximately 30 minutes at a time for full cardiovascular benefit.

Sport can extend skills you've already obtained from regular exercise – for instance if you enjoy swimming, why not join a water polo team or a swimming club?

The competitive element of sport encourages people to excel, but be careful not to become obsessed with winning. The bad sports who refuse to lose graciously may find themselves without a team.

If you're the type who bottles up feelings and sits on anger, try a game where you can really smash a ball around. Squash can be wonderful for letting out aggression.

If you are prone to back pain, avoid weight lifting, judo, jogging, violent squash and all contact sports, especially rugby; stick to exercises such as swimming, roller skating, cycling and walking.

Remember to do a warm-up with stretches before rushing out to take part in any sport, and a cool-down routine afterwards.

SPROUTING

Sprouted grains and seeds are an excellent and cheap source of protein, minerals, carbohydrates, and vitamins. They're crunchy, munchy and tasty too!

Sprouting increases the nutritional value of seeds and grains. Wheat, for instance, contains 30 per cent more vitamin B when germinating than its dormant grain. Try them in salads, with yoghurt or cottage cheese. They can be stir-fried, too.

How to sprout pulses and seeds

You need a few clean glass jars to act as sprouting containers, some gauze or cloth to cover the jars and some pure bottled water. Use alfalfa, adzuki, mung beans, lentils, fenugreek beans or chickpeas.

1 Soak the beans or seeds you are to sprout for 18 hours in pure water. The beans should have enough water so that they can 'drink' as much as possible.

2 Pour off excess water and place the drained beans in a warm, dark place. Cover the open jar with a cloth to prevent any debris falling in.

3 Rinse the beans twice a day, but ensure they do not stand in water, as this can allow moulds to grow.

4 Once sprouted, leave on a window sill in the sunshine for a few hours before eating.

Most beans, eg mung beans, chickpeas, lentils, take three to five days to sprout. Seeds like sunflower, sesame and pumpkin, take only one to two days.

STEAM

Throw bunches of fresh herbs – rosemary, parsley, marjoram and basil – into a bowl of boiling water. Lean over and put towel over head and around bowl. The steam will oxygenate skin cells, cleanse, hasten skin renewal and increase circulation. The heat opens the skin's pores, making cleansing easier. For that special occasion steep fresh blooms of roses, irises, or marigolds in the water. Cleanse afterwards with a gentle cleansing lotion, splash face with cold water and moisturise thoroughly. Steaming before using a face mask will make the treatment more effective. (See MASKS.)

Steam inhalations are particularly effective for respiratory problems. Add one or two drops or any of the following essential oils – basil, benzoin or myrrh, sandalwood, thyme or eucalyptus and use as above, inhaling for ten minutes. Repeat up to three times a day.

Steam baths have been enjoyed for centuries to draw out the body's toxins and reduce fluid. But anyone with high blood pressure, diabetes or heart disease should give them a miss.

Steam can be used effectively in your kitchen. It is the most nutritious way to cook vegetables, and preserves flavour as well as vitamin and mineral content. Steamers can be bought from most shops selling kitchen utensils and are an invaluable investment for anyone wanting to get the most out of their diet.

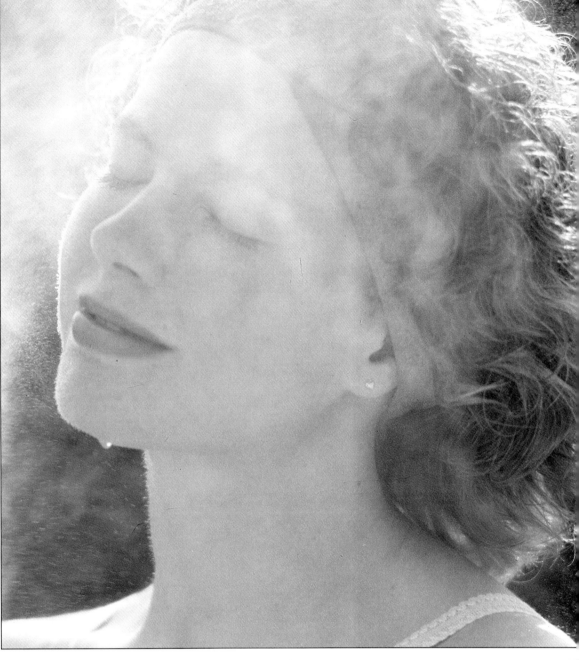

STRESS

In manageable doses stress is stimulating, challenging and motivating. It's when stress in our lives becomes so great that we feel unable to cope that it threatens our mental, emotional and physical well-being. It robs our body of essential vitamins and minerals, triggers high blood pressure and fatigue, distorts our skeleton causing back pain, aching joints and muscles and is a factor in most prevalent diseases.

When we are under stress the body responds immediately: adrenalin flows; the liver releases blood sugar into the bloodstream; heart rate and blood pressure rise to prepare for the activity to come; stomach juices cease flowing and the contractions of the intestine and other tubular organs cease so that no energy is wasted on unnecessary activity; the pupils of the eyes dilate; the mouth goes dry; the neck and shoulder muscles tense automatically; sweating starts and breathing become more rapid.

This state of alert worked wonderfully when life was simpler for humans. When attacked we would either run away or fight. If we needed food, we hunted or perished. If our body's response to stress was poor, we died – so an efficient response to stress ensured the survival of the fittest.

However, the fight or flight option is not appropriate to 20th-century life. Our bodies are more likely to go into a state of alert in response to bills, overdrafts, traffic wardens, rows with partners, crying children, traffic jams, bereavement, house moves, or divorce. A fight or flight response doesn't deal effectively with these problems.

If we are under permanent stress, the body does not function in a normal manner, and our general health is quickly affected.

There are skills and strategies you can incorporate into your life to stop stress taking control of you:

● **Learn to compensate:** if you hit a spell when things are going badly at work or at home, compensate by putting energy into those areas of your life which are still under your control. This may be the time to start redecorating a room, learn a new sport or improve your social life.

● **The art of delegation:** don't try and do everything yourself, either at home or at work. You will eventually run yourself into the ground and become irritable and unpleasant to be with.

Boredom: for some there seems too much time. Boredom creates its own stresses. Do not allow yourself to stagnate – make an effort to seek new experiences and challenges, and mix with interesting and stimulating people. Don't sit around waiting for things to happen, make them happen!

Building self-confidence: periods of stress create feelings of self-doubt. These thoughts can easily run away with themselves so that you begin to doubt even your ability to cope with simple problems. Bolster your self-confidence by recalling problems you have dealt with successfully in the past. Seek out friends who can be positive with you and reassure you. Make a list of your positive characteristics. This is no time to be modest; your ability to survive stress in your life depends on your ability to retain a positive attitude towards yourself.

Plan for stress: don't adopt a firefighting attitude and react to problems as they arise. Many potentially stressful situations can be anticipated. Use your BIORHYTHMS and self-knowledge to anticipate times you may be less well able to cope with busy and potentially stressful days. Plan the most effective ways to deal with the problems which are likely to arise – remember to allow for times when you can switch off with relaxing interests, friends, sports.

Learn to say no: you can't do everything and no one should expect you to. If saying 'no' is difficult try assertiveness training.

Relationships: in times of difficulty there is often a tendency to withdraw from other people. But sharing problems can give a new perspective and possibly show you ways of solving them. Who knows you well enough to know when you are under stress, and do you listen to that person? Bad communication can cause a great deal of unnecessary stress – work at improving personal relationships. (See EMOTIONS, COUNSELLING.)

Personal balance sheet: we all like the status that winning brings, but success demands a price as well as bestowing rewards and you must judge your own balance sheet. Where are you going and why? Who are you trying to seek approval from? Is it yourself, your peer group, your parents? *You* have to approve of yourself before anyone else does.

Relax: Learn simple RELAXATION and MEDITATION techniques. Use deep BREATHING exercises.

SUGAR

Sugar is a most important energy supply. It comes in many different shapes and guises, some of which are better than others.

Sugar is a CARBOHYDRATE. Foods containing complex carbohydrates release their sugar load gradually over a longer period of time. This slow release makes them a much better source of stamina and continued energy.

Even though all carbohydrates ultimately end up as simple sugars, not all sugars have the same effect on the blood sugar level. As well as glucose and fructose food sugars, there are three other types known as disaccharides: maltose, sucrose and lactose.

Glucose is the fastest-releasing sugar and makes the blood sugar level shoot up very quickly. Fructose, found mainly in fruit, is the next fastest.

The effect that different types of sugars have on your blood sugar level can be measured. When sugar enters the bloodstream, blood glucose levels rise. The pancreas then releases insulin which helps to transport the glucose from the blood into the cells. The result is a decrease in blood sugar levels. (Diabetics do not produce enough insulin to hold down glucose levels and 30 per cent of diabetics in this country need insulin injections.)

Refined sugar is sugar beet which has been stripped of its vitamins, minerals and natural fibre. It is a major cause of tooth decay, and medical evidence shows that over-consumption can raise the level of blood fats, contribute to atherosclerosis, and place stress on the pancreas.

A diet high in refined sugar adds on the pounds, too. Even so, we manage to eat about two pounds a week of the stuff. Any food containing complex CARBOHYDRATES or naturally rich in fructose and vitamins or minerals is far more healthy than refined sugar.

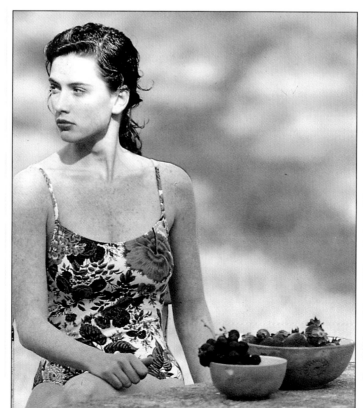

You needn't be concerned about how much sugar your diet contains as long as you avoid refined sugar as much as possible and don't drink too much concentrated natural sugar in pure fruit juice. Make sure you eat plenty of fresh fruit, beans, peas and pulses. If you do need sugar for taste, try raw, brown sugar. It's only the real thing if it still contains the thin film of molasses surrounding the sucrose crystal. The darker the sugar, the richer it is in nutrients.

There are a number of sugar substitutes such as xylitol, glycoside, fructoses, saccharine and cyclamates. They should all be taken in moderation and preferably as part of a programme to cut out added, refined sugars from your diet.

SUN

There's nothing lovelier than a sunny, spring day – it boosts our energy, warms our bodies and brightens our moods. We get up earlier and smile more often when the sun's around.

Sensible doses of sunlight are essential for our well-being. It triggers a series of chemical reactions which creates vitamin D in our bodies

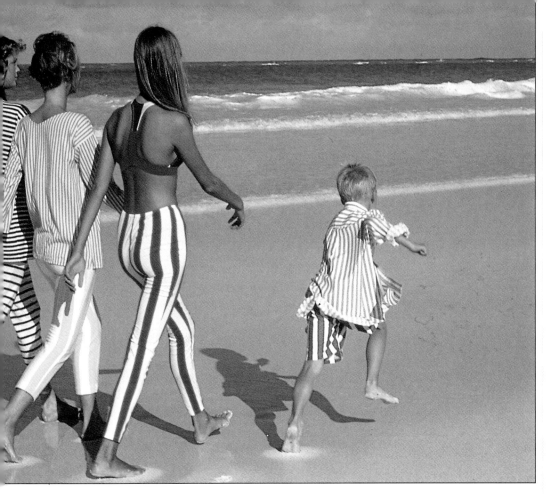

for the proper absorption of calcium and phosphorus – essential for strong bones and teeth (see OSTEOPOROSIS). Light skin patches on black skin can indicate a lack of vitamin D – supplement with cod liver oil and a vitamin D-rich diet. Sunlight can also regulate irregular menstrual cycles. Research shows that sunlight entering the eyes has some effect on the pituitary gland which helps regulate hormone production and that, unlike our ancestors who spent more time out of doors, we are not exposing ourselves to a health-promoting amount of light.

Don't spend all day indoors. Get out as much as you can, not just for lungfuls of fresh air, but for the light – especially if you're suffering from jet lag or irregular periods.

But remember, the sun's rays can be harmful. For why and how, see ULTRAVIOLET RAYS.

SUPPLEMENTS

Vitamins and minerals are essential for good health, so it is important to maximise your natural intake, as well as being aware of the areas where you might need to supplement your diet. It's better to develop the habit of balanced eating than to rely on taking supplements.

A balanced diet will give you protein, carbohydrates, fats and fibre, plus vitamins and minerals in the right proportions. Every day you should include a good mix of the following foods – fresh fruit, vegetables, wholegrain products, wheat bran, wheatgerm, pulses, dairy products, fish oils, lean meat in small quantities, and plenty of water.

Never exceed the recommended dose of any supplement without medical advice and take only for a short period until you look and feel better. Your body can often tell you whether or not you need supplement . . .

Puffy eyes – probably deficient in vitamins A and C. Take a multivitamin tablet with added C. Increase your intake of citrus fruits, green and yellow vegetables.

Black circles under the eyes – could be anaemic or maybe your body is retaining toxic wastes. Drink plenty of water and eat lots of liver, raw vegetables (especially spinach) and fruit. Iron tablets or iron tonic may be needed.

Oily hair – could be a hormonal imbalance. Try taking lecithin or a multivitamin tablet containing lecithin and zinc. Cut down on fat in your diet. Eat fresh green vegetables.

Dry hair – possibly a vitamin B deficiency. Try taking B complex tablets and eat plenty of brown bread, green vegetables, liver and nuts.

More colds than usual? Take vitamin C in powder or tablet form. Eat lots of citrus fruit and drink plenty of fresh orange juice. Eat potatoes with their skins on.

You may also need supplements if you:

Smoke – vitamin C.

Drink lots of coffee – vitamin B, potassium, zinc.

Eat a lot of junk/processed foods – multimineral tablets (bound in protein for easier absorption), cod-liver oil, brewer's yeast, powder or tablet form, lecithin, iron. (See JUNK FOODS.)

Drink ALCOHOL in excess – vitamin B complex, mineral supplement, evening primrose oil.

Take the contraceptive pill – Vitamin B6, B12, B1, C and E.

Are highly stressed – vitamin B complex, vitamin C.

Are menopausal – calcium tablets with vitamin D. (See OSTEOPOROSIS.)

Have symptoms of PREMENSTURAL SYNDROME – vitamin B6, magnesium and evening primrose oil.

(See DIET, VITAMINS, EVENING PRIMROSE OIL, MINERALS.)

TEARS

In ancient Rome, women kept two delicate glass phials – one for each eye. They collected their tears in them and when full, handed them to their husbands who then had to make recompense.

Tears are symbols of our sorrows, but we can cry with happiness, too. The saline, clear liquid which falls from our tear ducts is not only a way of expressing emotion, but also washes and cleans our eyes.

Expressing tears is healthy. A good cry that leaves cheeks wet and eyes red and swollen, but clear, is an indication that pent-up emotions have been released. There's a wholesome feeling of pure relief – like the aftermath of rain on a scorching hot day.

Research shows that people who cry easily are more able to resist infection and suffer less from stress-induced disease. Tears are an indication of emotional health – but very often childhood conditioning makes it difficult for us to show our emotions. Crying in public or with others makes us feel weak and vulnerable and we tend not to do it unless overwhelmed. Men particularly suffer from this repression. If you can't express your feelings through crying, either in company or alone, you may need to seek COUNSELLING to help you overcome major emotional blocks.

TEETH

Teeth are tough. Here's the proof – if a tooth was heated up alongside a steel ballbearing, the bearing would melt long before the tooth had even altered.

A healthy tooth stuck on the end of a drill, so that it hit aluminium or brick head on as the drill went through, would remain unmarked.

Feel how your teeth grip as powerfully as any pliers and crush or grind as effectively as a grinding machine 50 times their size.

Most people's teeth in this country aren't able to live up to their natural toughness because they are damaged in the first 15 years of their life by acid. The enormous amount of sugar consumed by the average Briton feeds the bacteria in our mouths which produces the damaging acid. It eats into the tooth's thin outer layer of enamel and infects the soft dentine underneath, producing that nagging toothache.

But it isn't tooth decay which mainly threatens our teeth. It's gum disease. A staggering 90 per cent of us suffer from gingivitis or gum disease without even realising it. If your gums bleed when you brush your teeth or you suffer from BAD BREATH, your gums are suffering and you could lose your teeth.

Plaque is the main culprit. Sticky films of food and bacteria accumulate between teeth and if this isn't removed the neglected bacteria will attack gums. If you want to hang on to your teeth, make sure you brush them every day and increase your intake of vitamin C, which is believed to reduce the risks of gum infection.

Chewing on apples, raw carrots, hard pears or celery will not only provide some of the vitamin C you need but will also stimulate and massage the gums. Always use dental floss between the teeth – it reaches the nooks and crannies a toothbrush can't. Cut out sugar.

Poor calcium intake in babies, growing children and menopausal women will weaken the teeth. Milk, dairy products, kelp, brazil nuts,

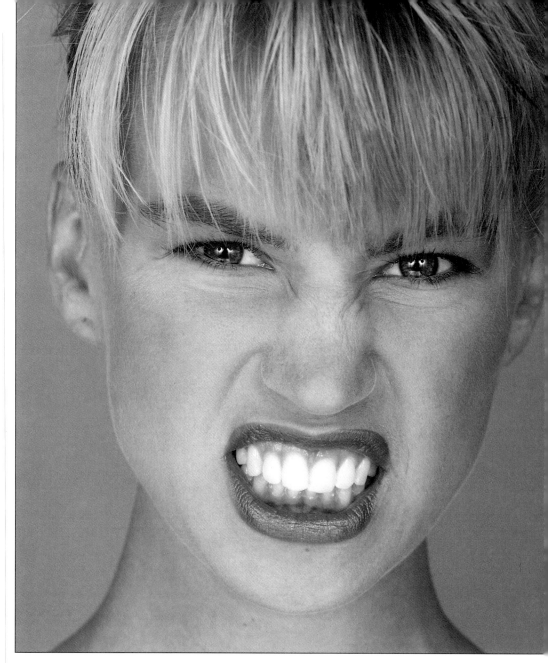

According to the British Health Dental Foundation, this is the best way to clean teeth ...
● Start with the upper jaw, place brush on gum and sweep brush to tips of teeth with a rolling action of the wrist – just as you would sweep away crumbs from your lap
● Make sure you include the backs of your teeth. Work your way round the upper jaw not forgetting outside edges of back teeth, then move onto the lower jaw.
● Brushing should take at least five minutes – look in the mirror and get to know your mouth
● Finish off with dental floss to reach the spaces a brush can't.

almonds, tinned salmon, tinned sardines, turnip greens, tofu, yoghurt and soya beans all contain calcium. (See OSTEOPOROSIS.)

Brushing your teeth at least twice a day and after meals is essential if your teeth are to spend the rest of their life with you (see left).

The main point of brushing is to rid your teeth of the film of plaque that normally builds up during the day. It allows sugar acid to feed off it and damages teeth.

Regular and efficient brushing helps prevents tartar accumulation between the teeth and gums, which eventually loosens teeth. Tartar is formed from the calcium that is naturally carried in your saliva and is a bit like the furring of a kettle. Brushing should take at least five minutes, and if you want to check

whether you've reached all those nooks and crannies, suck a disclosing tablet. It colours plaque bright red and is easily rinsed off.

The shape of your toothbrush is less important than the way you use it – a small nylon head of medium stiffness is generally recommended.

Your teeth are more precious than diamonds – keep them that way!

TEMPERATURE

The normal temperature of the human body is around 98.4°F or 37°C. This fluctuates quite normally from slightly lower in the morning to higher in the evening.

Your body's temperature is controlled by a centre in the brain co-ordinating the number of ways the body can regulate its own heat, such as sweating to lower your temperature, or by shivering to produce heat from the muscles.

Temperature can indicate whether or not a sick person is deteriorating and whether extra care needs to be taken. A thermometer gives the most accurate temperature reading. Make certain it has been washed thoroughly in soap and warm water before using. Shake sharply (holding the non bulbous end) so that the level of mercury is below 96°F. Place bulb end under the tongue, close mouth. Wait for three to five minutes. Don't hold thermometer while waiting.

With small children place thermometer under armpit and wait for five minutes.

Babies need a rectal reading – the

most accurate. Insert lubricated end of thermometer no more than 2.5cm (one inch) into the back passage. Leave in place for two minutes. Gently hold the baby's ankles together to keep buttocks closed.

Fever is a sign that the body is fighting infection, but should not climb higher than 103°F (39.5°C). Give plenty of liquids to prevent dehydration and sponge neck, forehead, arms and legs with tepid water. Do not dry skin. If temperature does not lower, call a doctor. Note any other symptoms such as vomiting, red or dull eyes, rashes.

Temperature can also indicate whether or not a woman is ovulating – daily temperature-taking is part of natural birth control, along with noting changes in cervical mucus.

THALASSOTHERAPY

Thalassotherapy is another way of pampering your body, mainly with sea water. This form of therapy is particularly popular on the Continent and includes fierce jets of water aimed at the body to revitalise muscles and stimulate the circulation.

Seaweed and essential oils are important aids to the water treatments. For instance, a mineral-rich seaweed cream is painted on the body, and then washed off once the vital nutrients have been absorbed into the skin.

If the body is wrapped tightly in bandages that have been treated with a mixture of seaweed and algae, the body's intake of iodine, calcium and magnesium is believed to be increased – particularly beneficial for cellulite.

THIGHS

Thighs in this country are mostly hidden under skirts and trousers. It's when we take them off at the sports centre or on the beach that you notice all is not well with British thighs. They tend to be flabby, CELLULITE-prone and weak.

It doesn't have to be that way, as regular exercisers know; both men and women can have firm, sleek thighs at any age.

If the thought of outdoor EXERCISE of any kind gives you the shivers, get an exercise bike, set it up in front of the television and cycle while you view. Do this three times a week through your favourite programme and you'll be suprised at the improvement! Climb stairs at every

opportunity rather than get into a lift, and if you have stairs at home practise stepping up and down on the first step, or run up and down 15 times. You might find your carpet wearing out, but your thighs will firm up and gain extra strength and stamina.

Swimming, cycling, running, walking are all excellent thigh conditioners.

MASSAGE thighs gently after exercise – it's surprising how tense the inner thighs, in particular, can get. Use a little light massage oil such as almond. And if you've an eye on seduction, add three drops of a fragrant essential oil. Try rose for women and jasmine for men.

THREAD VEINS

Thread veins are capillaries, those very fine blood vessels immediately below the skin. If they become more noticeable than usual, as red blotches on the skin, they are often described as broken, though this is not always the case. More usually they are 'stretched capillaries'. Capillary walls are elastic and dilate when the skin is hot, or in response to certain foods and alcohol, and then contract to their normal size again.

But for some people capillaries are permanently dilated, either on the face or on their legs. This can be due to a diet which includes lots of spicy food, alcohol, coffee and strong tea, circulatory disorders or extreme changes of temperatures.

Camomile, parsley and rose are all essential oils which, if added to a light carrier oil such as almond and gently massaged into the skin twice a day, will help restore the elasticity of the capillaries. But improvements may not be seen for at least six months.

Sclerotherapy is the main form of treatment for broken capillaries. A sodium sulphate-based liquid is injected into the surface of the skin and into the capillaries, causing them to shrink and fade. Each treatment lasts from 30 to 45 minutes and most people need up to four treatments. There tends to be bruising for up to three weeks, during which time legs or face should not be exposed to the sun.

Electrolysis can remove veins in the face, but when used on the legs can lead to scarring.

Any treatment is useless unless all stimulants such as alcohol and coffee are cut out from your diet, and hot baths are avoided along with saunas and other steam treatments.

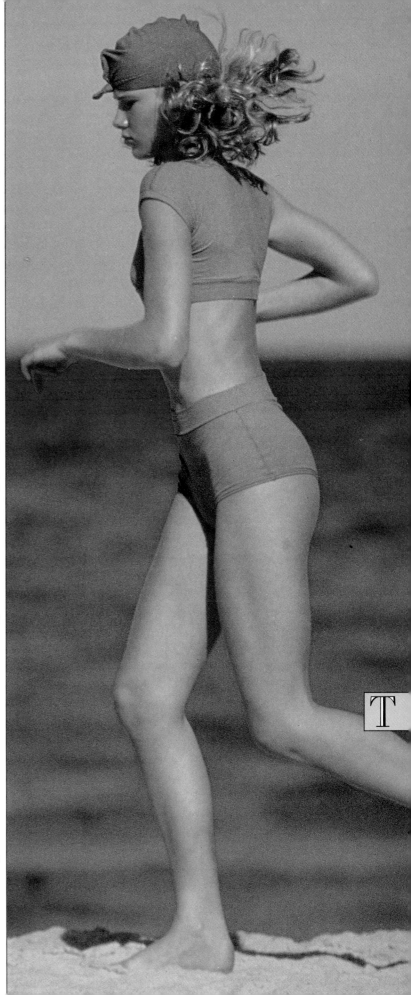

T

THRUSH

Thrush is an infection of mucous membrane by the fungus known as candida albicans. It may sometimes affect the mouth, but is most often a vaginal infection.

Everybody has candida organisms in their body, and in normal conditions they are prevented from flourishing by intestinal flora.

The vagina has a built-in defence mechanism in the form of beneficial bacteria, some of which take the glucose from the vaginal wall cells and transform it into lactic acid, creating an acidic environment. Unfriendly bacteria require a sweet, alkaline climate to reproduce.

Many factors can upset the balance including sex, bubble baths, tight trousers, tights, emotional upset, semen, antibiotics, the contraceptive pill, lack of sleep, diabetes, pregnancy, menopause and menstruation.

Try adding anti-fungal essential oils to your bath water if thrush is a problem. Myrrh, lavender or Ti-tree can be mixed together or used separately. Or add half a cup of vinegar to the bath. Yoghurt tablets, or lactobacillus capsules can be taken to help restore the vaginal flora. Eat plenty of live yoghurt, too.

If thrush is a recurring problem, wear loose skirts/trousers and cut down on your sugar intake. Drink water only, avoid yeast and cut out dairy products. Wine, fruit juices, tea and coffee can aggravate thrush.

If one partner has thrush, the other should be checked for the infection.

TONGUE

The surface of the tongue is more sensitive than the fingertips. Apart from its special sense of taste, the tongue has very finely tuned senses of touch and temperature. This sensitivity is due mainly to minute projections (papillae) from the tongue's surface, which give it a velvety texture.

Our ability to taste is thanks to taste buds grouped into specific areas. They detect single tastes such as sweet, sour, salt or bitter. Taste is also linked with the sense of smell.

The tongue itself is mainly muscle stretching back to the base of the skull below the ears. These muscles mould themselves with remarkable precision to meet the requirements of eating and speech.

Food particles, dried mucus and bits of the tongue's covering tend to accumulate on the tongue's surface. Normally it's cleared by saliva but the tongue can become coated or furred if saliva is reduced because of fever, not enough liquid intake, or loss of appetite. The tongue is sensitive to deficiencies of iron and some vitamins. A sore tongue indicates anaemia due to lack of iron and vitamin B12 (see VEGETARIAN, VEGAN.)

When brushing the teeth, always gently brush the tongue too. It clears its surface of any debris and helps fight bad breath. Rinse the mouth thoroughly afterwards.

In Chinese medicine the tongue is believed to be an offshoot of the heart and to have direct links with the body's 12 vital organs. Seventeenth-century Chinese herbalists and acupuncturists observed the balance of Qi – the life force – in these organs by examining the tongue.

The first consideration is the colour of the tongue which is sometimes described as the tongue's 'spirit'. A healthy tongue is vibrant, pale red and 'fresh', indicating a healthy body. It should be supple and stable when stuck out and should be neither swollen nor too thin. It should also be ulcer-free.

Normal tongue coating is thin and white, indicating the healthy functioning of digestion, and is thicker at the root of the tongue than at the tip.

A pale, swollen tongue that is slightly too moist indicates a weakness of the digestive system. Symptoms include acute tiredness and feeling cold much of the time.

A pale, slightly dry, thin tongue is believed to indicate a blood deficiency, resulting in menstrual problems, poor memory, insomnia, tiredness and lethargy.

A dry, red tongue with a yellow coating can indicate emotional problems such as repressed anger, resentment manifested by headaches, constant thirst, constipation and poor sleep patterns, including bad dreams.

A very red, uncoated tongue with a crack in the centre can hint at stomach and kidney problems, possibly caused by poor or irregular diet and a deficiency of certain vitamins.

The alcoholic's tongue tends to be dark purple and distended, with a thick coating.

Tongue screening is used as a complementary aid in Chinese diagnosis along with face colour, pulse, skin texture and abdominal palpation.

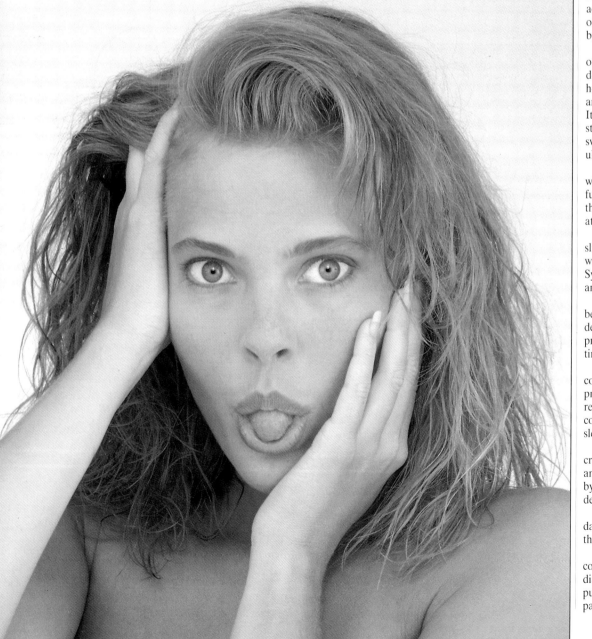

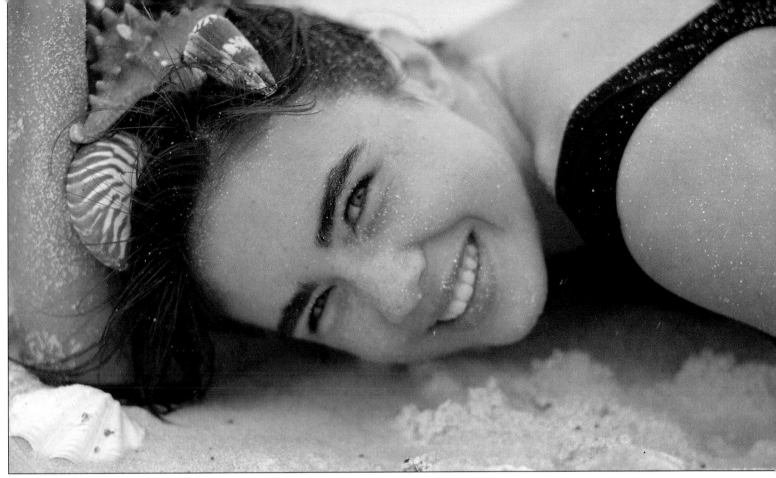

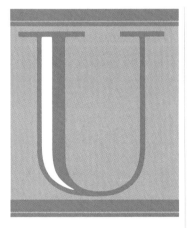

ULTRAVIOLET RAYS

Light includes ultraviolet wavelengths of UVA, UVB and UVC. UVB rays are the ones that tan us and are likely to burn. UVAs reach deeper into the skin and are linked with cancer and ageing, while UVC rays are screened by the earth's atmosphere.

A tan is a protective reaction to the harsh rays of the sun. The production of melanin, the skin's natural pigmentation, is triggered by ultraviolet rays to prevent us from burning. Dark, olive skins and black skins produce more melanin than the fair, Celtic type of skin. No suntanning lotion can give a tan of a specific depth, whatever the package promises. The colour of your tan will depend entirely on the amounts of melanin your skin can produce.

Safe and successful tanning – that won't leave you looking like a shrivelled prune and at risk to skin cancer – depends on your choice of sunscreen and careful acclimatisation to the sun's rays.

The most effective sunscreens contain one of the B-complex vitamins, para-aminobenzoic acid – PABA for short. It prolongs the time you can spend in the sun. (It can also cause an allergic reaction – skin becomes rough, red and itchy, but can be soothed with hydrocortisone cream containing no higher than one per cent hydrocortisone.)

Sunscreen products are usually graded with a Sun Protection Factor (SPF) indicating how long you can stay out in the sun. For instance SPF4 means you can stay out in the sun for four times as long as the time it would take you to burn had you not applied sun protection. Unfortunately there is no internationally uniform method of estimating SPF. Rely on knowing your skin type and the strength of the sun at your holiday's location.

For sensitive skin of the type associated with redheads and freckles, dermatologists recommend sunscreens with a high SPF, preferably 15. Fair skins shouldn't spend more than ten minutes between 11am and 3pm in the heat, and dark skins should aim for a maximum of 20 minutes during the first day of exposure to the sun. Remember that melanin takes three days to build up in your skin and be fully effective.

If you have oily, spot-prone skin use a non-greasy gel or oil-free lotion. Try a cream or milky lotion for normal to dry skins. Reapply after spending time in water, and every 80 minutes if possible – but this doesn't extend the SPF, the time you can spend in the sun.

A WINTER TAN

Regular stints in a solarium not only accelerate a tan, they also accelerate the ageing of the skin. The artificial ultraviolet light in a solarium can emit more than ten times the radiation of the summer sun at high noon. The effect on your skin is cumulative – the more exposure you get, the greater your chances of developing WRINKLES, discoloured patches of skin and eventually skin cancer.

Don't wear perfumes, make-up, or deodorants while using a solarium, as certain chemicals can burn or irritate the skin when exposed to intense ultraviolet light. Don't use a solarium if you are on antibiotics, as this could also cause a skin reaction.

Always wear goggles in the

FIVE SOLAR POWER POINTS

UV passes through clouds

Altitude increases the strength of UVB rays. Every 3,000 metres (10,000 feet) above sea level adds four per cent to the burning effect of the sun

Reflection boosts solar power. White surfaces, snow, water and sand reflect UV rays. Direct sunlight can also penetrate water to a depth of five metres (16 feet) and can easily burn skin

The sun is at its most powerful around midday. Don't sunbathe between 11am and 3pm. It's possible to burn even in the shade at midday

It is always high summer at the equator

IF YOU BURN...

Soak in a tub of cool water

Afterwards apply cold wet towels to painful area

Splash cider vinegar on sunburned skin. Rub lightly on to burned area

Smooth on vitamin E ointment

solarium. Over-exposure of the eyes to ultraviolet light can burn the cornea and result in permanent eye damage.

If it's a blush of colour you're looking for during a drab winter, why not try a vigorous EXERCISE programme or even a ten-minute stint in a SAUNA twice a week instead? These will stimulate circulation and give your cheeks a healthy vibrant glow – naturally!

HAIR CARE
Hair suffers from ultraviolet rays, too. Exposing unprotected hair to the strong summer sun bleaches and discolours it, and dehydrates the hair's structure.

Hair that has been chemically treated is particularly vulnerable. Bleached hair can become slightly green when exposed to strong sunshine plus the chemicals used in swimming pools.

If you want to keep your hair gleaming and lustrous while still making the most of the holiday sun, try some of the following tips:
⬤ Don't apply oil to hair that is exposed to the sun – the effect is like frying.
⬤ Protect your hair by wearing a scarf or sunhat whenever possible.
⬤ Take a deep-conditioning hair product on holiday with you. Apply when having a siesta.
⬤ Use a protective hair shield gel with UV screens.
⬤ If possible, braid hair, or tie into a pony tail or top knot. This reduces the surface area exposed to sun.
⬤ Wear a swimming cap in pools to protect hair from chlorine.

U NDERWATER MASSAGE

Underwater massage isn't what it suggests. It isn't a deep-sea diver complete with flippers, goggles and oxygen tank massaging you several fathoms below.

It's administered in a larger than average bath filled with warm water. The tap end looks rather like a car dashboard with various dials and indicators, and the masseur directs a pipe at your body and adjusts the pressure of the water which gently massages you.

This is an excellent way to stimulate a sluggish lymphatic system and helps budge CELLULITE. The jets of water break up deep muscular tension in a way that a hand massage can't – it would be too painful. The bathwater lessens the

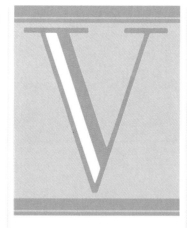

V ACUSAGE

This is a form of electrical massage treatment. A series of plastic cups are placed on the skin and slid to the nearest lymph node, where all toxins are released. Vacuum suction massage is believed to improve circulation and help in the reduction of fatty deposits. It is often used in conjunction with slimming treatments to reduce hips and thighs. (See MASSAGE.)

V EGAN

Vegans follow a form of vegetarianism which uses no animal produce at all. A vegan diet not only excludes meat and fish but also all dairy products and eggs.

This restricts sources of protein even more than the usual vegetarian diet and makes the inclusion of alternative protein-rich foods such as nuts, seeds, beans and lentils crucial.

The lack of dairy products in a diet seriously restricts calcium intake. Natural sources of calcium include almonds, brazil nuts, molasses, turnip greens, tofu, soya beans. There is also a danger of deficiencies in VITAMINS D, E, B12, zinc and especially iron.

See VEGETARIAN for ways to boost these nutrients without eating meat and fish.

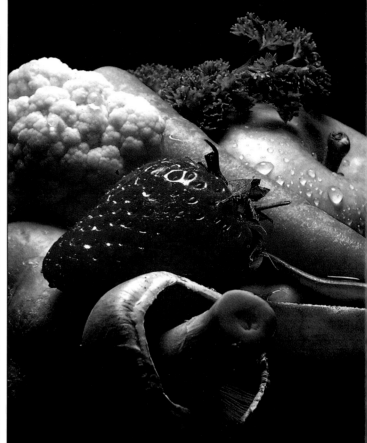

V EGETARIAN

Approximately 1.5 million people in Britain don't eat fish or meat, and the number of vegetarians is increasing rapidly.

Vegetarianism is not a modern fad – the Greek mathematician Pythagoras was vegetarian.

If you are contemplating becoming a vegetarian either because you don't like the idea of animals being killed for food, and/or for health reasons, make sure you balance your diet so that the VITAMINS, AMINO ACIDS and MINERALS that are lost through not eating meat are replaced.
⬤ Fat soluble vitamins A, D and E are high in animal produce because they can be stored in the animal's body. Increase your intake of green, leafy vegetables, and carrots and beetroots to compensate. Vitamin D is made in the skin by sunshine and should be taken as a supplement either in liquid or capsule form during the winter. Vitamin E is found in almonds, apricot oil, corn oil, hazelnuts, margarine, sunflower seeds, walnuts, wheatgerm, wholewheat flour.
⬤ Animal produce is only a marginally better source of protein than nuts and seeds. Soya beans and

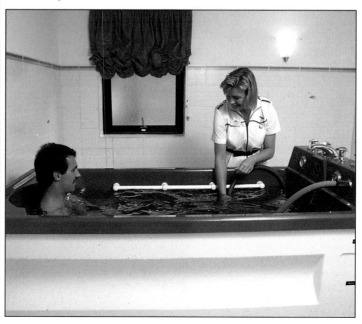

milk provide more protein than meat, so increase your repertoire of bean dishes, and step up brown rice intake. Both beans and rice are also high in complex CARBOHYDRATES and FIBRE – you are improving your diet in more ways than one. Eggs provide a small amount for protein, and also make up for a lack of some essential AMINO ACIDS, particularly isoleucine and lysine.

● Meat contains plenty of iron in easily digestible form, so make sure you're replacing it by eating plenty of iron-rich foods (spinach, milk, eggs, wheatgerm, walnuts, wholegrain products, seaweed, pumpkin seeds). Vitamin C increases the absorption of iron – a glass of orange with a boiled egg, for example, can increase iron absorption fivefold.

● Vitamin B12 promotes growth and development, treats pernicious anaemia, promotes metabolism of fat and carbohydrates and maintenance of normal function of nervous system. As it is not found in vegetables, vegetarians commonly suffer from a B12 deficiency. It is found in milk and eggs, Swiss cheese and blue cheeses. If you don't like dairy products, you may need to take it in as a supplement. Signs of B12 deficiency include appetite loss, profound fatigue, sore tongue, poor memory, yellow eyes and skin, and bleeding gums. Supplements can be taken in oral or injectable forms until sympton of deficiency have cleared.

If you think vegetarian food is bland, try this tasty classic.

VEGETABLE LASAGNE
Serves 6
1lb lasagne
8oz soya beans, cooked
2 onions, chopped
8oz mushrooms, chopped
1 clove garlic
½ green pepper, chopped
2 stalks celery, chopped
3 tbs chopped parsley
14oz-can tomatoes
1 vegetable stock cube
1 bay leaf
¼ tsp thyme
¼ tsp oregano
2 tsp sugar
Salt and pepper
1lb cheddar cheese, grated
1lb cottage cheese
Parmesan cheese
Preheat oven to Gas mark 5 (190°C, 375°F). Grease large baking dish. Sauté beans in oil with onions, mushrooms, garlic, pepper, celery and parsley until soft. Add tomatoes, stock, herbs, sugar and seasoning. Simmer for 15 mins.

Cook lasagne as per packet

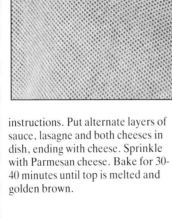

instructions. Put alternate layers of sauce, lasagne and both cheeses in dish, ending with cheese. Sprinkle with Parmesan cheese. Bake for 30-40 minutes until top is melted and golden brown.

VINEGAR

Vinegar was always kept in our grandmothers' kitchens, not just for culinary purposes but as a traditional remedy for a variety of minor ailments. For instance . . .
For sore throats
● A tablespoon of cider vinegar mixed with hot water and honey makes a soothing drink. Taken twice a day it acts as a cleansing medicine.

● Gargle with a mixture of malt vinegar, salt or sodium bicarbonate in warm water.
● Inhale steam from vinegar diluted with four times its volume of boiling water.
For varicose veins
● Apply neat cider vinegar to veins at night and in the morning. Leave the vinegar to dry on the skin.
For genital thrush
● Add half a cup of vinegar to a warm bath.
For sunburn
● Dab on cider vinegar.
For healthy hair
● Add a few teaspoonfuls of malt vinegar to the rinsing water after shampooing. If you're a brunette, this will bring out the natural highlights in your hair.

VISUALISATION

Imagery and visualisation are techniques that are being increasingly used by both cancer and Aids patients, but they have wide implications for ill health generally.

Imagery in cancer was first used in America and involves imagining a cancerous tumour, for example, being attacked and cleaned up by the body's defence system. For instance, you visualise white blood cells as fish swimming about eating up grey cancer cells. The image is projected as if you were watching it on a screen in your mind's eye. At this point you become one of the fish and lead the rest into attack. You feel yourself as the fish eating. At the end of each visualisation you picture yourself at the healthiest time in your life and create images of the present with you feeling as you did then.

An essential component of visualisation is the faith and belief that you will get better. It can be used in many ways. Some people find the visualisation of 'attack' too aggressive and war-like. Images should be adapted to whatever suits the individual. For instance, the body can be seen as a garden, and the visualiser gives water and nourishment to the plants and banishes the weeds.

Visualisation is not easy, and the big danger is that patients who do not feel they are getting anywhere will feel a failure. It's best to speak to a teacher who is able to feed an image into your conscious and unconscious mind (in much the same way as a hypnotist).

Visualisation should not be seen as a cure, although there are claims that it can and should always be combined with other treatments. It may suit some people, but not others. But it's worth trying, so next time you have a cold or a sore throat, imagine…

VITAMINS

Vitamins are chemical compounds vital for growth and health. Some vitamins form essential parts of HORMONES, others are essential for the efficient use of enzymes (chemical molecules that facilitate the completion of chemical reactions).

In a well-balanced diet of food grown in nutritionally adequate soil (see GREEN), there should be a supply of the most important vitamins. But there are times and habits, such as smoking, when vitamin supplements may be needed. (See SUPPLEMENTS.)

Vitamins are divided into two separate categories.

VITAMIN	SOURCES	FUNCTIONS
A fat soluble	Found in carrots, root vegetables, sweet potatoes, spinach, cheese, milk, eggs, apricots, liver and fish oils.	Protect from infections, help growth and repairs tissues, good for healthy eyes.
B1 (thiamine) water soluble	Found in wholemeal bread, brown rice, pulses, yeast extract, cornflakes, meat, peanuts, bran.	Promotes growth, essential in metabolism of carbohydrates, improves brain and nerve function.
B2 (riboflavin) water soluble	Found in fish, eggs, milk, yeast.	Aids growth and reproduction, healthy eyes, skin, nails and hair.
B3 (niacin) water soluble	Body makes its own. And from poultry, nuts, grains, fish, eggs, liver, yeast.	Helps regulate blood sugar and cholesterol.
B5 (pantothenic acid) water soluble	Found in grains, yeast, eggs, green vegetables, liver, molasses, brewer's yeast, chicken.	Aids adrenal gland, energy production and immune system.
B6 (pyridoxine) water soluble	Found in wheatgerm, bananas, turkey, yeast, eggs, wholegrain cereal, offal, beef, milk.	Essential for protein manufacture, production of red blood cells and antibodies.
B12 (cyano-cobalamin) water soluble	Found in meat, eggs, milk, cheese. And body makes its own.	Essential for cell life, healthy nervous system, metabolism of iron.
C (ascorbic acid) water soluble	Found in green, leafy vegetables, potatoes, tomatoes, fruits, berries.	Functions vital for many body functions including wound and disease healing. Extra C required by smokers or those under stress.
D fat soluble	Made by body from sunlight, fish, dairy foods.	Enables proper use of calcium and phosphorus to build healthy bones.
E fat soluble	Found in vegetable oils, milk, eggs, nuts, eggs, dark green vegetables.	Protects circulatory system and cells, and retards ageing process. Fat soluble
K fat soluble	Green vegetables, turnips, cereals, egg yolks, yoghurt, alfalfa, fish oils.	Vital for blood clotting.

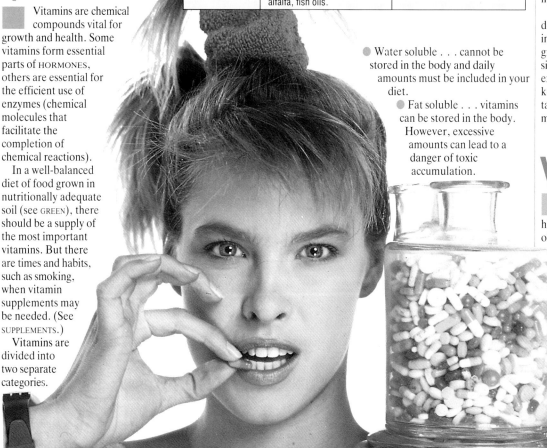

● Water soluble . . . cannot be stored in the body and daily amounts must be included in your diet.

● Fat soluble . . . vitamins can be stored in the body. However, excessive amounts can lead to a danger of toxic accumulation.

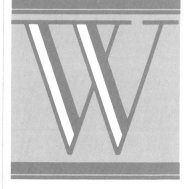

WARM UP

Before any exercise session you should warm up to prevent straining muscles. A warm-up session need last no more than five minutes and should include some general stretches and movement such as walking on the spot and swinging arms to stimulate circulation and motor nerves in preparation for safer, more effective functioning of MUSCLES.

Both your muscles and connective tissue will be nourished by the increased supply of oxygen via the blood and will become more supple. Preparing your body this way for strenuous exercise helps prevent ligament and tissue injury.

Equally important is the cool-down. After energetic exercise it is important to slow down your pulse gradually. Don't suddenly stand still, sit or come to a halt once your exercise session has stopped, but keep walking or jogging on the spot, taking deep, slow breaths for several minutes until your body feels calm.

WATER

An 11-stone man has about 42 litres (74 pints) of water in his body. Approximately two-thirds of the water found in our bodies is held within cells, while the remaining third travels around our body in our blood and other fluids.

We can lose up to 25 litres (44 pints) of fluid during the day through the amount of water vapour we lose through breathing and sweating, as well as through excretions.

It is important to drink at least 2 pints (1.1 litres) of water each day – excluding that used in other drinks – to replace what is known

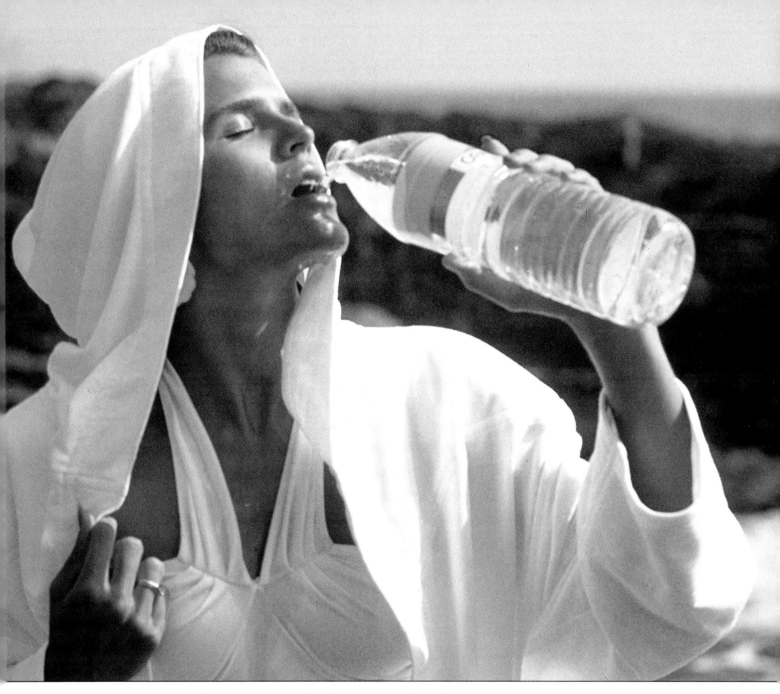

as 'the obligatory loss', but aim to drink a minimum of four pints (just over two litres).

If the level of the body water drops below a certain level, you will feel dry, thirsty and weak. You will generally feel thirsty after exercise or heavy manual work. As you exercise, more water is lost as you sweat and also as you breathe. The concentration of salt in the blood increases and if you don't drink to rebalance your body's loss, you'll start to feel lethargic.

It's difficult to drink too much water – the extra fluid helps flush out the body's toxins and dilutes urine, which if too concentrated can cause kidney stones and cystitis.

Pure water can be the best health drink to accompany a balanced, wholesome diet. But tap water may contain pollutants, particularly in urban districts where it is reprocessed several times.

● It is estimated that 17 per cent of people in England and Wales will receive tap water which breaks at least one parameter of the EEC drinking water directive. In East Anglia, Lincolnshire, Nottinghamshire and Staffordshire over a million people receive water with concentrations of nitrates from agricultural fertiliser over the EEC limits. (See GREEN.)

● Always use the cold tap for drinking and run the tap for a few minutes in the morning to flush out stagnant water.

● Fit a filter to your drinking-water tap and follow instructions carefully, or drink bottled mineral water – it contains potassium, calcium and magnesium in the small amounts the body needs.

● Check that you don't have any lead pipes. If, for any reason, you are concerned about your tap water, arrange to have a sample analysed by your Water Authority.

WATER WORKOUTS

Working out in water is a wonderful way to strengthen and tone muscles. You don't even have to be able to swim! You weigh only ten per cent of your body weight in water, so physical strain is reduced to a minimum – great for those with bad backs and/or extra weight, and the pregnant, arthritic and unfit.

Bob around to warm up before exercising and between exercises if water gets chilly. And always end your pool workout with a low bob. Here's how to get your body bobbing…

Stand chest deep in water and jog on the spot. Your movements will be slower than on dry land because the water will be resisting you. Hold on to the side of the pool at first, then move further out. Keep bobbing until you feel warm and are a little out of breath.

Now you're ready for the top-to-toe toning exercises shown on the next page.

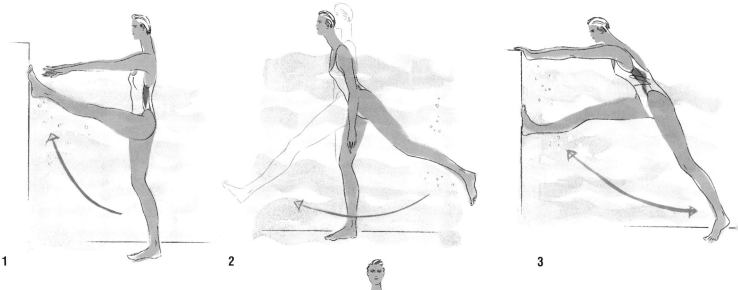

1

2

3

Try these exercises in your local swimming pool…

1 Hand-toe touch
Stand upright with ankles together and arms stretched in front of you at shoulder height. Keeping legs straight, kick left leg up to left hand. Lower, then repeat with right leg. Repeat 12 times.

2 Leg lift
Hold on to side of pool with right hand, right arm at right angle to poolside. With feet apart, raise left leg as high as possible, then swing back as far as possible. Turn around and repeat exercise with right leg. Repeat 12 times.

3 Leg stretch
Grip the wall with both hands, keeping arms straight. Raise right leg to touch wall, with left leg stretched back. Keep arms straight and level with surface top of water. Change leg positions quickly. Repeat 12 times.

4 Thigh and hip exercise
With heels together and middle back against wall of pool, raise right leg as high as you can, then pull leg across front of your body and back again. Alternate legs. Repeat 12 times.

5 Abdominal exercise
With both hands on the pool rail, tuck up to a backstroke start position. Keeping arms straight, kick back with both legs together, so you're lying full length in the water. Lower one arm to steady yourself against wall if necessary. Tuck up again. Repeat 12 times.

6 Arm rowing
Stand in water with feet about two

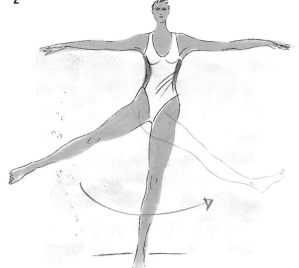

4

5a

5b

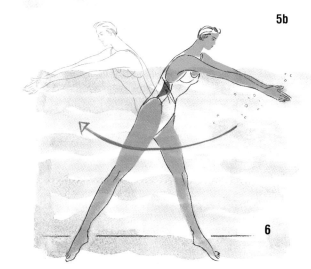

6

feet apart. Link hands together to form a large paddle and swing arms from side to side. Repeat 12 times.

7 Hip rotation
Stand in water with feet apart at hip width. With hands on hips, look upwards and rotate the hips in a large circle.

8 Water jog
Stand in water, lift alternate knees, as if jogging on the spot. Twenty lifts each leg.

9 Arm rotations
Stand in water with both arms by your side, palms facing forwards. Bring arms up through the water, turn palms in and brush ears with upper arms, then continue circling arms back to starting position. Repeat 12 times.

10 Breast stroke and crawl
Holding on to edge of pool, tuck up and kick back legs. Lie on water, keeping arms straight. Do five breast stroke kicks, then five crawl kicks, legs straight and splashing feet up and down.

11 Ballerina leap
Stand in water with your right leg forward and left leg back. Raise right arm in front of you with palm down and left arm behind you with palm pointing up. With head above water jump to alternate position of arms and legs. Repeat 12 times.

12 Waist turn
With back against the side of pool, lay arms over the edge. Keep back and bottom against wall and raise both knees to chest height. Move both legs left then right. Repeat 12 times.

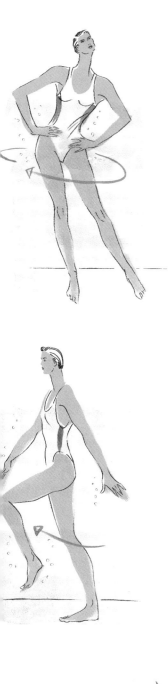

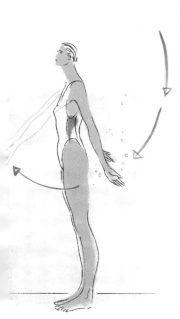

WAX

Waxing is an effective way to remove hair from legs and the bikini line. Its effects are not permanent and the process can be uncomfortable. It can be done in a salon or by yourself at home with various kinds of wax strips which are applied and then pulled off.

There are two ways of using wax to remove hair professionally. The method most frequently used involves applying cool wax with a spatula, placing thin strips of calico on top of the wax and pulling sharply away to bring off the hairs with the set wax. The process takes about 15 minutes for both legs, from ankle to knee.

With the second method, thicker wax is applied and then pulled off. This process is effective for coarse hair and takes about half an hour for both legs. Rub in an antiseptic cream afterwards.

Paraffin wax is sometimes used to ease stiff joints and rejuvenate the skin. Warm wax is applied to either the whole body or specific parts such as hands or feet. The wax is left for half an hour while you luxuriate in a lovely feeling of cosy warmth. The retained body heat encourages perspiration and may lead to weight loss. This type of wax treatment is not used to remove hair as the wax does not set in the same way and is peeled off slowly and gently.

WELL WOMAN CLINICS

Well Woman Clinics cover all types of health services for women. Some provide counselling and advice on emotional as well as health matters, while others may concentrate on only one area of health, such as cervical screening or contraception.

Well Woman Clinics can be private or NHS. Contact your local Community Health Council to find out more about your own local clinic and any HEALTH-CHECK services for men.

WRINKLES

'What? And erase 60 years of living!' retorted one famous actress when told she ought to have a face lift. She's right. Wrinkles give a face character.

Wrinkles occur because the connective tissues that form most of the inner layers of the skin, such as collagen, lose elasticity. Skin which is repeatedly stretched by the muscle contractions goes back to its original smooth state when young, but not as the connective tissue ages.

Excessive sunlight (see ULTRAVIOLET RAYS), wind and cold, harsh soaps and environmental POLLUTION all conspire to damage the skin, making it easier for wrinkles to form. It takes about 300 million contractions to permanently work a fold into your skin. Women's skin wrinkles faster than men's, mainly because their COLLAGEN is thinner and loses elasticity sooner.

The best protection against wrinkles is a good sunscreen applied daily to exposed skin, as well as moisturising cream or lotion. The ESSENTIAL OILS frankincense and neroli oil have been used in skin care for thousands of years and have a preservative action upon the skin. Add three drops of either to an egg cupful of almond oil and massage into the skin; leave until absorbed and cleanse.

But remember, smiling causes fewer wrinkles than frowning. If your wrinkles are where smiles have been, do you really want to wipe away the souvenirs of years of laughter?

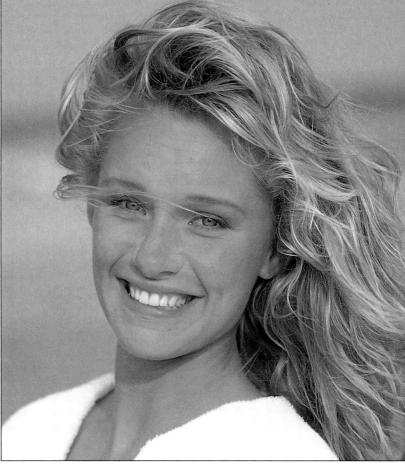

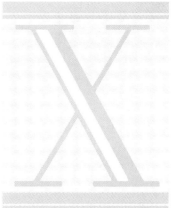

X CHROMOSOMES

The sex of a child is determined at conception. Both sperm and egg have 23 pairs of chromosomes – one of which is a sex chromosome.

The father determines the sex of the child; the sperm carries either an X or Y chromosome and the egg carries two X chromosomes.

If sperm carrying the X chromosome enters the egg there is an XX configuration – a girl. If sperm carries a Y chromosome the resulting configuration is XY – a boy.

X-rays are electromagnetic rays of very short wavelength which have so much energy they crash through living tissues like a bullet. They are stopped only by high density metals like lead.

The body absorbs a little of this radiation in proportion to the density of its tissues. In diagnosis, the shadows of the absorbed X-rays are recorded on special film, outlining soft tissues as well as bone.

A number of related diagnostic techniques use X-rays . . .

In fluoroscopy the X-ray shadow of the body is cast on a screen which can then be photographed.

A brain scanner uses a moving beam of X-rays to move across the brain and gradually build up a three-dimensional picture.

A contrast medium is often injected into the body to change the density of certain tissues in order to distinguish them in X-ray pictures. The medium can be air (injected into the brain cavities) or barium given as a meal or enema to observe the digestive system.

Most people are aware that diagnostic radiation can cause some damage. There is no safe dose below which X-rays are harmless.

The US Academy of Sciences has calculated that one barium examination of the intestines gives as much cancer risk as smoking five to 20 cigarettes each day for a year. A low-dose, dental X-ray is believed to be the equivalent to smoking half a cigarette daily for a year.

Avoid radiation where the benefits are just not worth the risks. If X-rays are used to look for internal injuries, broken bones or suspected serious problems such as a lump in the breast, they can be considered justified.

Before agreeing to an X-ray:
● Check there aren't previous ones that could be used.
● Ensure there is proper shielding – insist on a lead apron at the dentist. The testes and ovaries must be shielded.
● Obey instructions during the X-ray – you don't want to have to do it again.
● Ask whether or not the equipment has been recently serviced and inspected.
● Protect children – especially the unborn. Tell your doctor if you are, or may be, pregnant and avoid X-rays unless the doctor thinks it essential and safe. Young children

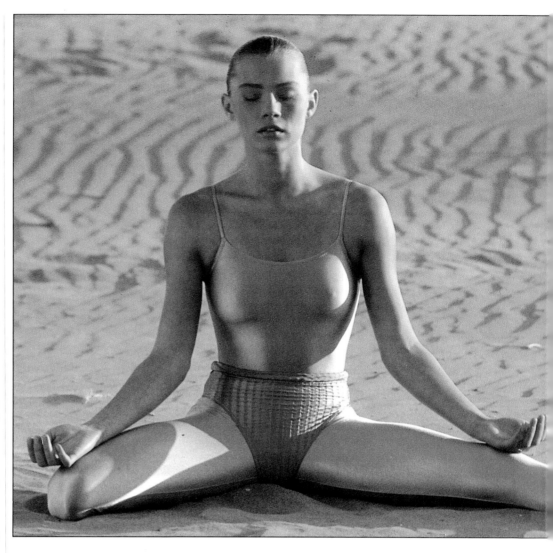

are particularly vulnerable to the carcinogenic nature of X-rays, so make sure they are always properly shielded.

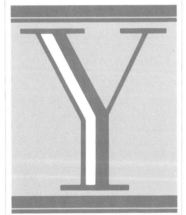

YOGA

Yoga evolved in India at least five thousand years ago, a system of Hindu philosophy showing the means of freeing the soul by concentrating the senses inwards, away from external objects. It deals with every aspect of physical, spiritual and mental health. No one is excluded from its benefits; it can be practised by people at all ages and stages of life and is taught both in classes and individually.

Yoga has a great therapeutic value and can prevent, cure and manage a wide range of disorders including digestive, musculoskeletal and nervous conditions.

Yoga literally means 'union' – the joining of the individual soul with the Divine or Absolute. But you don't have to be connected with any religious belief to practise yoga.

It is above all a way of maintaining health and preventing disease by correcting imbalances in the body before they have a chance to develop into serious health problems. In yoga the physical body is seen as a vehicle, the mind as the driver, and the soul as the true identity.

There are various schools of yoga but Hatha yoga is the most widely practised in the West.

Concentrating on simple stretching, breathing and relaxation exercises, Hatha shares the basic yoga belief in *prana* – a subtle form of energy permeating the world. Similar to the *chi* energy in ACUPUNCTURE and the healing energy of the West, prana flows along channels known as *nadis* (equivalent to the meridians of acupunture) and is concentrated in centre of energy called *chakras* which are dotted around the body.

Blockages of prana are believed to cause ill health, and the *asanas* (physical postures) act as purifiers of the body allowing the energy to flow freely.

It is best to learn yoga with an experienced teacher. Once you have learned the basics, you can then tailor your daily yoga routine to suit your own needs. Some yoga positions benefit certain mental and physical conditions and should be incorporated into your daily yoga exercises if needed.

(SEE MEDITATION, RELAXATION.)

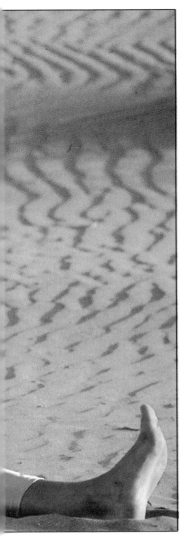

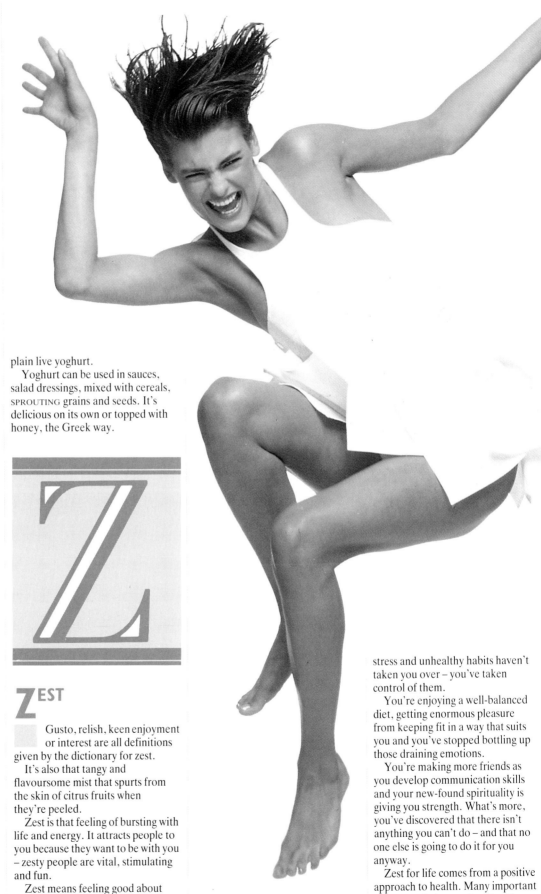

plain live yoghurt.

Yoghurt can be used in sauces, salad dressings, mixed with cereals, SPROUTING grains and seeds. It's delicious on its own or topped with honey, the Greek way.

YOGHURT

It is important to use only natural live yoghurt in your diet as this contains a cocktail of bacteria including lactobacillus and acidophilus that keep the intestines clean. Yoghurt also contains B-complex vitamins and vitamins A and D, so is excellent for maintaining clear skin. Used as a face MASK, either on its own, mixed with a little honey or blended with various fruits or tomatoes, it has a pleasant, softening effect.

Natural live yoghurt is helpful in the treatment of intestinal problems. If you are on a course of antibiotics, eat plenty of yoghurt both during the course and for a while afterwards. This will redress the bacterial balance of the intestines upset by the antibiotics, which can kill helpful bacteria.

Avoid commercially-sweetened yoghurts – they are likely to contain preservatives and additives and provide little of the advantages of

Z

ZEST

Gusto, relish, keen enjoyment or interest are all definitions given by the dictionary for zest.

It's also that tangy and flavoursome mist that spurts from the skin of citrus fruits when they're peeled.

Zest is that feeling of bursting with life and energy. It attracts people to you because they want to be with you – zesty people are vital, stimulating and fun.

Zest means feeling good about yourself, because you're in control of your life. It's positive proof that

stress and unhealthy habits haven't taken you over – you've taken control of them.

You're enjoying a well-balanced diet, getting enormous pleasure from keeping fit in a way that suits you and you've stopped bottling up those draining emotions.

You're making more friends as you develop communication skills and your new-found spirituality is giving you strength. What's more, you've discovered that there isn't anything you can't do – and that no one else is going to do it for you anyway.

Zest for life comes from a positive approach to health. Many important elements of a happy, healthy life are a matter of choice – *your* choice.

Z

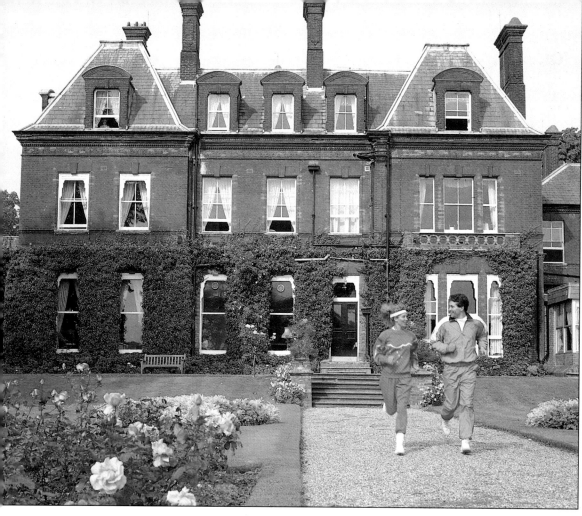

THE POSITIVE APPROACH TO A NEW LIFESTYLE

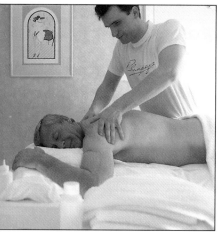

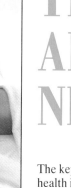

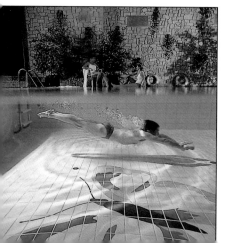

The key to a positive approach to health is achieving and maintaining a high level of physical and mental well-being. Look at a healthy person and you will notice an obvious enthusiasm for life, look further and you will find that a balanced lifestyle is second nature to them. Overall health doesn't come from dabbling in theories, thinking about weight loss one week, vitamins another, positive thinking another with the odd spurt of exercise thrown in when the weather is fine. Positive health stems from awarding yourself a lifestyle from which physical and mental well-being flows naturally.

Champneys Health Resort is dedicated to encouraging an enthusiasm for health and fitness which becomes part of every day life. It is a place to recharge and regenerate, to shed bad habits like smoking, drinking too much, eating junk food and working too hard. A dedicated team of Doctors, Dieticians, Exercise Instructors, Lifestyle Consultants, Beauty Therapists and other specialists are all committed to helping guests achieve and maintain a high level of physical and mental well-being for their lifetime.

If this conjures up a vision of a spartan existence in gloomy surroundings, think again. Champneys is set in 170 acres of parkland, a large, luxurious country retreat where tranquility reigns alongside a variety of social and leisure activities and extensive facilities.

Champneys first opened in 1925, the very first health resort of its kind in England. The key to its success is the Champneys' philosophy, we firmly believe that good health and the steps to achieving it can, and should be, fun. Champneys will help you to establish correct eating habits, to lose weight if necessary and to break destructive eating patterns. You can stop smoking, reduce your alcohol intake, discover the benefits of regular exercise and learn how to manage stress by developing relaxation techniques. You will be shown how to make the very most of your natural appearance and how to approach life with optimism. Above all, you will be individually encouraged and pampered and, since Champneys is unique in its field for its medical bias, your programme of good health will be tailored specifically to your needs. A huge range of treatments are available with separate facilities for men and women, plus a magnificent indoor swimming pool, gymnasium fitted with first-rate equipment, squash and tennis courts. There is a whole spectrum of daily activities, including body blitz classes, water exercises, yoga, morning stretch, backcare and relaxation courses, cycling, guided walks to explore the surrounding countryside and a complete programme of lectures, demonstrations and workshops. The mood at Champneys is that of a friendly country house, an atmosphere maintained by staff and guests alike and the emphasis is on informality and relaxation.

All the rooms are comfortably and tastefully decorated and flair and imagination is an essential part of the wholesome, delicious food service in the two restaurants, whether or not you choose to follow a strict dietary regime. Champneys is enjoyed by men and women of all ages, from busy executives to mothers taking a break from the children, from office high flyers to grandparents. Champneys will show you how to incorporate health and fitness into your way of life.

CONTRACEPTION – CHOOSE WITH CARE

	HOW DOES IT WORK?	HOW IS IT USED?	ADVANTAGES	DISADVANTAGES	WHAT ELSE?	HOW GOOD IS IT?*
COMBINED PILL	Synthetic oestrogen and progestogen hormones prevent release of egg. Also thickens cervical mucus and alters womb lining, so making it less likely to accept egg.	The pill is taken regularly on a 21, 22, or 28 day basis, depending on which type.	Doesn't interfere with intercourse. Tends to make bleeding lighter. Premenstrual tension may lessen. May protect against cancer and reduce risk of fibroids.	Side effects. Risk of clotting. May increase blood pressure. Some research links Pill use and cancers of the breast, cervix and liver. No STD protection.	Not for smokers and women over 35. See doctor every six months – sooner if you are worried. Effectiveness can be reduced by some medications including antibiotics.	99%
CONDOM	Prevents ejaculation of sperm into the vagina and possible fertilisation of egg.	Rubber sheath placed over erect penis. Must be held in place when penis is withdrawn immediately after ejaculation.	Readily available. Easy to use. Good back-up method. Prophylactic–protects against STD, Aids, HIV.	May break under pressure, can slip off and leak. Can interfere with sexual pleasure and spontaneity.	Essential if penetration is to be a part of safe sex. Can be part of foreplay. Weakened by air, light, heat.	85–98%
DIAPHRAGM (CAP)	These are barrier methods which fit inside a woman's vagina preventing sperm getting through to join an egg.	Vaginal diaphragms kept in shape by a pliable metal rim covered in rubber, fit over cervix. Cervical caps are smaller and fit neatly over cervix. Both used with spermicide.	Used only when needed so suitable for irregular sex. No side effects. Caps may protect against cervical cancer. Works as soon as it is in place. Some STD protection.	Can interrupt lovemaking. Spermicide can be messy. Cystitis is a problem for some users. Can take time to learn to insert.	First fitting must be by doctor. Don't use mineral or vegetable oil based spermicides. Insert cap well in advance of lovemaking and nearer the time top up with spermicide.	85–95%
INTRA-UTERINE DEVICE	Made of plastic with coating of thin copper wire and one or two soft threads attached.	Inserted into the womb via the cervix (neck of womb). The IUD is inserted (and removed) by a doctor.	Does not interrupt lovemaking. Suitable for women who have had children and for older women. Can be left for three to five years depending on type.	Can be expelled. More likely to get infection in womb and fallopian tubes. Can cause heavy periods. Possibility of ectopic pregnancy. No STD protection.	Check threads after each period. Have annual check ups. Never try to remove an IUD yourself.	96-99%
MINI PILL	The mini pill contains progestogen only. It thickens cervical mucus. The lining of the womb is less likely to accept a fertilised egg.	Must be taken same time each day. Take the first pill of the first pack on the first day of your next period. You will be protected at once.	Doesn't interfere with intercourse. Can be used by older women. Suitable for breastfeeding women.	May cause irregular bleeding. Risk of ectopic pregnancy – but rare. See GP immediately if you have sudden abdominal pain.	See your doctor at regular intervals. Ovarian cysts are common in mini-pill users, but usually disappear when pill is stopped. No STD protection.	98%
NATURAL METHODS	Aim to predict when woman is most fertile so that intercourse can be avoided at this time.	Fertile periods are worked out by daily recording of body temperature and by noting changes in cervical mucus, known as sympto-thermal method.	No side effects. Couples share responsibility for family planning. Become more aware of how bodies work.	Much care needed by both partners. Careful record keeping needed.	Must be learnt from a specially trained teacher. Can use barrier method during fertile time.	85–93%
SPERMICIDES	Form barrier between cervical opening and sperm. Chemical component (usually nonoxynol-9) coats and breaks down surface of sperm.	Foam is the most effective and is sprayed into vagina. Jellies and creams are used only with diaphragms and caps.	Vaginal lubricant. Provides some STD protection. Can be used during breast feeding. Good for infrequent lovemaking.	Not effective if used alone. Must be used at right time – all but foam require waiting period. Some spermicides cause vaginal discharge.	Use foam, jellies, creams as back-up for other forms of contraception.	75%
SPONGE	A soft circular polyurethane foam sponge inserted in vagina. Contains spermicide.	Placed in vagina and over cervix up to 24 hours before lovemaking and must be left in for six hours afterwards.	Remains effective for 24 hours One size fits all. Thrown away after removal. Some STD protection. No fitting required.	Should not be used during period. Not available from GPs.	Available from chemist. Expensive. Instructions for insertion and use can be learned quickly.	75-91%

* FPA figures

ADDRESSES

ACUPUNCTURE
The Acupuncture Association & Register,
34 Alderney St,
London SW1V 4EU.
Tel: 01-834 1012

ADDICTION/DEPENDENCY
Release, 169 Commercial St,
London E1 6BW.
Tel: 01-377 5905

AIDS and HIV
Terrence Higgins Trust,
52-54 Gray's Inn Road, London
WC1X 8JU.
Tel: 01-242 1010 – Helpline.
National Aids Helpline,
0800 567123 Freefone

ALCOHOL
Alcoholics Anonymous,
PO Box 1, Stonebow House,
Stonebow, York YO1 2NJ.
Tel: 0904 644026

SOCIETY OF ALEXANDER TEACHERS
10 London House, 266 Fulham
Road, London SW10 9EL

ALLERGIES
Action Against Allergy,
43 The Downs, London
SW20 8HG. Tel: 01-947 5082

ANOREXIA & BULIMIA NERVOSA
Anorexic Aid,
The Priory Centre, 11 Priory
Road, High Wycombe, Bucks
HP13 6SL

AROMATHERAPY
International Federation of
Aromatherapists,
44 Eastmearn Road,
London SE21 8LS

BEAUTY
British Association of Beauty
Therapy and Cosmetology,
Suite 5, Wolseley House, Oriel
Rd, Cheltenham, Glos

BREASTS
Breast Care & Mastectomy
Association,
26a Harrison Street, London
WC1H 8JG. Tel: 01-837 0908

COLOUR COUNSELLING
Color Me Beautiful
66 Abbey Business Centre,
Ingate Place, London SW8 3NS
Tel: 01-627 5211

Living Colours,
33 Lancaster Grove,
London NW3 4EX

MEDICINE
Institute for Complementary
Medicine,
21 Portland Place,
London W1N 3AF.
Natural Medicines Society,
Edith Lew House, Back Lane,
Ilkeston, Derbyshire DE7 8EJ

COSMETIC SURGERY
British Association of Plastic
Surgeons,
Royal College of Surgeons,
35-43 Lincoln's Inn Fields,
London WC2 3PN

COUNSELLING
British Association for
Counselling,
37a Sheep Street,
Rugby, Warks CV21 3BX.
Tel: 0788 78328/9

EXERCISE
Physical Education Association,
c/o North East London
Polytechnic, Lonbridge Road,
Dagenham, Essex RMS3 2AS.
Tel: 01-590 6149

The Sports Council,
16 Upper Woburn Place,
London WC1H 0QP.
Tel: 01-388 1277

GREEN
Friends of the Earth,
26-28 Underwood Street,
London N1 7JQ.
Tel: 01-490 1555

HAIR
Institute of Trichologists,
228 Stockwell Rd,
London SW9 9SU.
Tel: 01-733 2056

HEART
British Heart Foundation,
102 Gloucester Place,
London W1H 4DH.
Tel: 01-935 0185

HERBALISM
National Institute of Medical
Herbalists,
41 Hatherley Road,
Winchester, Hants SO22 6RR.
Tel: 0962 68776

HOMOEOPATHY
British Homoeopathic
Association,
27a Devonshire Street,
London W1N 1RJ.
Tel: 01-935 2163

Society of Homoeopaths,
2 Artisan Road, Northampton
NN1 4HU. Tel: 0604 21400

HRT
The Amarant Trust,
14 Lord North Street, London
SW1P 3LD Tel: 01-222 1220.
Information Helpline:
0836 400190

HYPNOTHERAPY
National Council of
Psychotherapists and
Hypnotherapy Register,
1 Clovelly Road,
London W5 5HE.
Tel: 01-840 3790/567 0262

National Register of Hypnosis
and Psychotherapy,
12 Cross Street, Nelson, Lancs
BB9 7EN. Tel: 0282 699378

IRIDOLOGY
National Council and Register
of Iridologists (NCRI),
80 Portland Road,
Bournemouth BH9 1NQ.
Tel: 0202 529793

British School of Iridology and
The British Register of
Iridologists,
Sheraton House, Castle Park,
Cambridge CB3 0AX.
Tel: 0223 462244

MEDITATION
Transcendental Meditation,
Freepost,
London SW1P 4YY.
Freephone 0800 269303

MELANOMA
Health Line.
Tel: 01-980 4848 (Ask for any of
over 200 tapes on health.)

OSTEOPATHY
British and European
Osteopathic Association,
6 Adelaide Road, Teddington,
Middlesex TW11 0AY.
Tel: 01-977 8532

London School of Osteopathy,
110 Lower Richmond Road,
Putney, London SW15 1LN.
Tel: 01-788 1991

OVERWEIGHT
Weight Watchers UK Ltd.
11 Faircacres, Dedworth Road,
Windsor, Berks.
Tel: 0753 856751

PREGNANCY
National Childbirth Trust,
Alexandra House,
Oldham Terrace, Acton,
London W3 6NH.
Tel: 01-992 8637

British Pregnancy Advisory
Service,
7 Belgrave Road,
London SW1.
Tel: 01-222 0985

Women and Medical Practice;
Health Information Centre,
666 High Road,
London N17.
Tel: 01-885 2277 (Offers a
register of alternative health
practitioners.)

REFLEXOLOGY
British Reflexology Association
Monks Orchard,
Whitbourne, Worcs WR6 5RB
Tel: 0886 21207

SHIATSU
Shiatsu Society, 19 Langside
Park, Kilbarchan,
Renfrewshire PA2 2EP

SMOKING
Action on Smoking & Health
(ASH),
5/11 Mortimer St,
London W1N 7RH.
Tel: 01-637 9843

VEGETARIAN
The Vegetarian Society UK Ltd
Parkdale, Dunham Road,
Altrincham, Cheshire WA14
4QG. Tel: 061 928 0793

YOGA
British Wheel of Yoga,
1 Hamilton Place, Boston Road,
Sleaford, Lincs NG34 4ES

GENERAL
Health Education Authority,
Hamilton House,
Mapledon Place,
London WC1H 9TX.
Tel: 01-631 0930
For general information on
preventive medicine

Please enclose large sae when writing for information.